Adhesive Restoration of
Endodontically Treated Teeth

Quintessentials of Dental Practice – 40
Endodontics – 4

Adhesive Restoration of Endodontically Treated Teeth

By

Francesco Mannocci
Giovanni Cavalli
Massimo Gagliani

Editor-in-Chief: Nairn H F Wilson
Editor Endodontics: John M Whitworth

Quintessence Publishing Co. Ltd.

London, Berlin, Chicago, Paris, Milan, Barcelona, Istanbul,
São Paulo, Tokyo, New Delhi, Moscow, Prague, Warsaw

British Library Cataloguing in Publication Data

Mannocci, Francesco
    Adhesive restoration of endodontically treated teeth. - (Quintessentials of dental practice; v. 40)
    1. Dentistry, Operative 2. Root canal therapy
    3. Prosthodontics
    I. Title II. Cavalli, Giovanni III. Gagliani, Massimo
    617.6'9

ISBN: 9781850971351

ISBN: 978-1-85097-135-1

Foreword

Adhesive materials and techniques, together with advances in fibre posts, have revolutionised the restoration of root canal treated teeth. This revolution offers many new exciting opportunities, but has created new challenges. *Adhesive restoration of endodontically treated teeth* – the latest, keenly awaited addition to the widely acclaimed *Quintessentials of Dental Practice* series, provides a concise, highly practical overview of modern principles and procedures for the restoration of root canal treated teeth in clinical practice. The information and guidance included in this volume is of immediate practical relevance.

If you are still using traditional approaches to restore root canal treated teeth, apply bonding procedures, but in a limited range of situations, or wish simply to better understand where, when and how to use fibre posts and associated materials, then this book should be a priority on your "must read" list.

For those who have already purchased and read volumes in the *Quintessentials* series, the format will be familiar – easy to read, authoritative text, accompanied by numerous high-quality illustrations, with each chapter concluding with carefully selected suggestions for further reading. All of this condensed into a book which takes only a few hours to read, with the prospect of a huge return for your time and effort. For many, the restoration of root canal treated teeth will never be the same again.

Another carefully crafted, well-illustrated volume, further expanding and enhancing the *Quintessentials* series – one of the most efficient and effective ways to learn about, understand and apply modern concepts and procedures in clinical practice.

Congratulations to the authors for a job well done.

Nairn Wilson
Editor-in-Chief

Preface

The restoration of root canal treated teeth has changed considerably in recent years. Dentine bonding systems, composite resins and fibre posts have largely replaced amalgam cores and cast metal posts; all-ceramic and composite crowns have superseded metal-ceramic crowns in the management of aesthetic problems. Many universities across the world are now teaching the use of fibre posts and composite as the principal means of restoring root-filled teeth.

Key advantages of contemporary adhesive techniques include:
• Immediate post-endodontic placement of a post and core build-up.
• Design and construction of the post-endodontic restoration under the direct control of the dentist.
• Securing an immediate and enhanced post-endodontic coronal seal.
• Provision of restorations with improved aesthetics.
• Ability to preserve and bond to tooth tissue which would be removed in conventional, non-adhesive techniques.

This is a book on adhesive restorations. As a consequence, other techniques are not considered in any detail. This does not mean that non-adhesive restorations such as Nayyar cores and cast metal posts are no longer valid modalities of treatment, but the evidence supporting the use of fibre posts and composite exceeds the evidence in favour of metal posts and cores.

The aim of this book is to provide the general practitioner with principles and techniques for the adhesive restoration of root canal treated teeth. Most of the techniques described in this book have been used and refined by the authors over the past 12 years; most of them have also been tested in two clinical studies published in peer-reviewed journals. As this is a practical book, the scientific evidence supporting our work is not described in detail. The reading lists contain references to relevant clinical and scientific data.

In addition to considerations of restoration placement, consideration is given to retreatment, including the removal of fibre posts, which may present special challenges for the general practitioner.

Discussion of the restorative decision-making processes is included in the concluding chapter, to be read subsequent to the description of the adhesive restorative options for the restoration of root canal treated teeth.

Francesco Mannocci
Giovanni Cavalli
Massimo Gagliani

Further Reading

Mannocci F, Qualtrough AJ, Worthington HV, Watson TF, Pitt Ford TR. Randomized clinical comparison of endodontically treated teeth restored with amalgam or with fibre posts and resin composite: five-year results. Oper Dent 2005;30:9–15.

Mannocci F, Bertelli E, Sherriff M, Watson TF, Ford TR. Three-year clinical comparison of survival of endodontically treated teeth restored with either full cast coverage or with direct composite restoration. J Prosthetic Dent 2002;88:297–301.

Acknowledgements

Many thanks to Nairn Wilson and Tom Pitt Ford for their continuing support and encouragement.

Special thanks to John Whitworth. This book would not exist without his help.

We would like to thank Luca Boschian, Andrea Felloni and Dario Mezzanzanica for their invaluable support, together with Riccardo Cantoni for his outstanding technical support in respect of the crown and bridgework illustrated in this book.

We would also like to thank Dr Keith Cohen for providing the implant images of Chapter 9.

Contributors

Bhavin Bhuva BDS, MFDS, RCS (Eng), MClinDent student in Endontology, King's College London Dental Institute at Guy's, King's College and St Thomas's Hospitals London, UK.

Giovanni Cavalli MDS, private practice, Brescia, Italy.

Laura Figini DDS, private practice, Milan, Italy.

Massimo Gagliani MD, DDS, Associate Professor of Endodontics and Restorative Dentistry, University of Milan, Italy.

Fabio Gorni DDS, private practice, Milan, Italy.

Francesco Mannocci MD, DDS, PhD, Senior Lecturer in Endodontology/Honorary Consultant in Restorative Dentistry, King's College London Dental Institute at Guy's, King's College and St Thomas's Hospitals London, UK.

Shanon Patel BDS, MSc, MClinDent, MFDS RCS (Eng), MRD RCS (Edin), Specialist Endodontist, King's College London Dental Institute at Guy's, King's College and St Thomas's Hospitals London, UK, and private practice, London, UK.

Contents

Chapter 1
The First Step: the Endodontic Treatment

Aim

To describe the principles of root canal treatment and their impact on the subsequent restoration of the tooth.

Outcome

After reading this chapter, the reader should have a clearer understanding of the role of microbial infection in periapical disease, the rationale for each stage of root canal treatment, and the importance of a suitable post-endodontic restoration. The reader should also appreciate the impact of each stage of root canal treatment on the subsequent restoration of the tooth.

Introduction

The purpose of root canal treatment is to prevent apical periodontitis in teeth with irreversible pulpitis and to heal apical periodontitis in teeth with infected, necrotic pulp spaces. Root canal treatment allows teeth to remain in healthy, pain-free function in the dental arch, and to justify confidence and expenditure in respect of a definitive long-term restoration.

The dentine–pulp complex is protected by a hard, impermeable outer casing of enamel. Once these barriers are breached by, for example, caries, operative dentistry, tooth surface loss or trauma, the underlying permeable dentine–pulp complex becomes susceptible to microbial, chemical and/or physical injury. Injury may occur as a result of noxious stimuli reaching the pulp indirectly via patent dentinal tubules, or directly if the pulp becomes exposed to the mouth. The pulp tissue within the root canal space will become inflamed and ultimately necrotic, allowing microbial infection to progress. Eventually, this will lead to the development of periapical disease.

Patients with pain of dental origin may present with signs of pulpitis or apical periodontitis. Once a diagnosis of irreversible pulpitis or apical periodontitis has been made, the tooth should be assessed according to the guidelines in

Chapter 8, and the treatment options of extraction versus root canal treatment and subsequent restoration discussed with the patient. When discussing treatment options, it is essential to advise that root canal treatment is not an end in itself, and that post-endodontic restorative treatment will be required to restore the tooth back to function and aesthetics. It should be stressed that the timing, nature and quality of the coronal restoration may have a critical bearing on endodontic success and tooth survival. Only then can an informed decision be made on the most suitable treatment for the tooth in question.

Stages of Root Canal Treatment

Root canal treatment can be broken down into stages:
- preoperative assessment and preparation
- preparation of the pulp space (including access and instrumentation/disinfection)
- sealing the pulp space
- provision of a sealing and protective coronal restoration.

Restoration should be considered as an integral element in the package of endodontic care.

The prognosis of endodontic treatment is dependent on a systematic approach. Each stage must be successfully completed before embarking on the next if consistently predictable results are to be achieved.

Preoperative Assessment and Preparation

Once the diagnosis has been confirmed, it is essential that the prognosis of the tooth is determined. Restorability must first be established, taking into account both the quantity, quality and location of coronal tissue, and the periodontal status. Carefully "walking" a periodontal probe around the gingival margin of the tooth will highlight the presence of significant features such as vertical fractures, which may have a serious impact on restorability and treatment planning. It is common for teeth that require endodontic treatment to be heavily restored or broken down and infected. Caries must be removed to prevent leakage and minimise the risk of microbe-laden carious dentine entering the root canal space during treatment (Fig 1-1).

Ideally, there should be a minimum of 2 mm of sound supragingival tooth tissue around the circumference of the tooth for subsequent restoration with a cuspal coverage restoration (Fig 1-2). If there is any doubt in respect to the

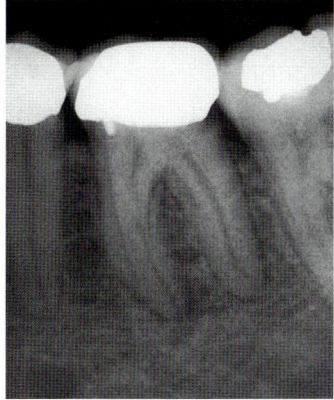

Fig 1-1 Radiographic signs of caries at the distal margin of a lower molar crown. The crown must be removed to fully excavate caries and assess restorability before root canal treatment can commence.

prosthodontic restorability (see Chapter 8), the existing restoration should be completely removed to reveal the extent and location of residual sound tooth tissue (Fig 1-3). It is essential to inform the patient and secure their consent prior to embarking on this type of exploratory treatment. If the tooth is found to be unrestorable, an informed decision should be made to extract rather than attempt a heroic restoration.

Complete removal of the existing restoration is advisable in a range of circumstances. This may reveal hidden fracture lines, which may not have been identified by external examination or periodontal probing (Fig 1-4).

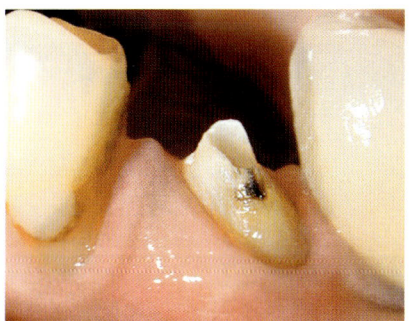

Fig 1-2 At least 2 mm of supragingival coronal tooth tissue should be present on all tooth surfaces for optimal restorative prognosis after root canal treatment.

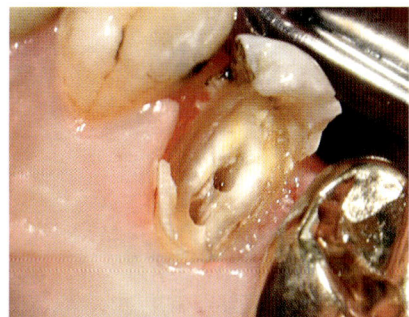

Fig 1-3 Removal of the failing restoration and caries revealed that this premolar tooth was unrestorable. It was extracted and replaced with an implant.

3

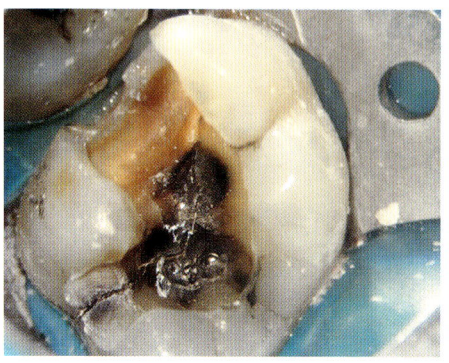

Fig 1-4 Fracture lines indicating that this tooth will require a cuspal coverage restoration very soon after endodontic treatment.

Such careful exploration may be time and effort well spent, determining not only the restorability of a tooth but also:

- The type and design of the post-endodontic restoration required.
- How soon after endodontic treatment a definitive restoration should be placed.
- Whether cusp reduction, the placement of a well-fitting copper ring, orthodontic band or a provisional crown is required to prevent cuspal fracture during and immediately after root canal treatment (Fig 1-5). Extracoronal support of this sort may also be required to allow a secure, well-sealing rubber dam to be placed.

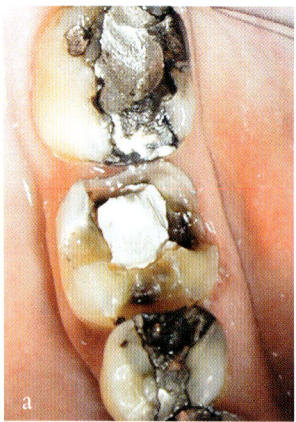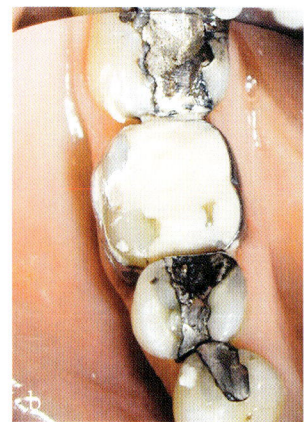

Fig 1-5 (a) Restorations in this lower molar tooth have been removed. (b) The remaining buccal cusps have been braced with an orthodontic band filled with a glass-ionomer cement.

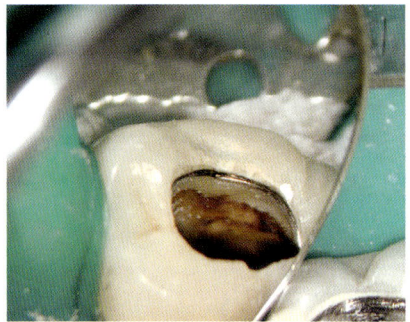 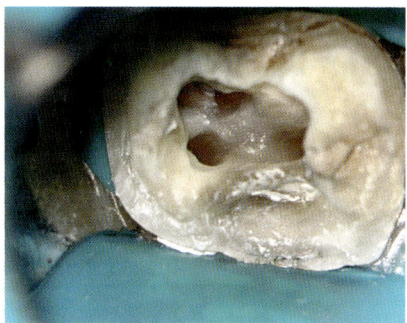

Fig 1-6 (a) Access cavity preparation in this lower molar has revealed a significant amount of caries which was not detected on preoperative radiographs. The crown must be removed for caries excavation and assessment of restorability.

Fig 1-6 (b) Removal of existing crowns assists in the location and preparation of canals.

Crowns must be removed prior to root canal treatment if significant coronal leakage or caries are suspected, or are detected once the tooth is accessed (Fig 1-6a). Root canal treatment can be more challenging if a decision is made to access the pulp through a crown, as the anatomical landmarks of the tooth may be masked by the extracoronal restoration. This may lead to difficulties in identifying the root canal entrances, the inadvertent removal of excessive sound dentine (Fig 1-6b) or even perforation. In all of these situations, the risks should be assessed and an informed decision made to remove the crown before treatment is commenced.

Even if, as a consequence, a decision is made to work through a crown, it is always wise to advise the patient that circumstances may dictate that the crown is removed during treatment and that a new crown may be required once the treatment has been completed.

Endodontic treatment must be carried out under a rubber dam (Box 1-1) (Fig 1-7). Good illumination and the use of magnification are essential to carry out root canal treatment to a consistently high standard. Similar conditions are also required for the stages of restoration using an adhesive approach.

Preparation of the Root Canal Space
Preparation of the root canal space can be divided into two stages; firstly, access cavity preparation and, secondly, instrumentation and disinfection of the root canal space.

Box 1-1 **Functions of a rubber dam**

- Protects the patient from risks of swallowing or inhalation of endodontic instruments and materials.
- Eliminates bacterial contamination of the root canal space from saliva.
- Prevents leakage of irrigants into the oral cavity.
- Improves visibility for operator by retraction of soft tissues (cheek, tongue).
- Improves comfort for patients.

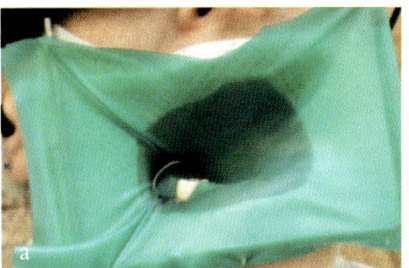
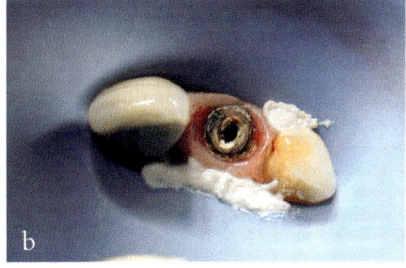

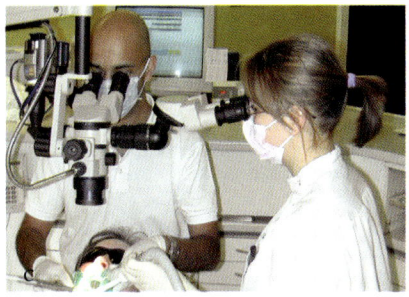

Fig 1-7 (a) A rubber dam is mandatory when carrying out endodontic treatment. (b) The split dam technique may be used to isolate teeth which cannot be easily isolated, OraSeal® is used to plug any gaps between the gingivae and rubber dam. (c) Good illumination and the use of magnification are essential.

Access cavity preparation

The aim of access cavity preparation is to identify the root canal entrances for subsequent instrumentation and disinfection of the root canal space. Access cavity preparation can be one of the most challenging and frustrating aspects of endodontic treatment, but it is the key to successful treatment. Inadequate access may complicate canal location and negotiation, and impact on the prognosis by compromising debridement, disinfection and sealing of the root canal space. It may contribute also to instrument separation and canal aberrations (e.g. transportation and ledging), which may impair infection control and ultimately lead to treatment failure.

It is unusual for access cavities to follow precisely the classic outline forms of young, previously unrestored teeth, as commonly illustrated in endodontic textbooks. The dimensions of the pulp chamber and location of the root canal entrances will be influenced by the amount and position of secondary and tertiary dentine deposition in response to caries, restoration, leakage and tooth surface loss over the course of a tooth's life. These cumulative insults may have a dramatic, and not necessarily chronological effect, on the size and shape of the pulp chamber (Fig 1-8a–c).

The objectives of access cavity preparation are to:
- remove the entire roof of the pulp chamber to allow the coronal pulp tissue to be eliminated
- produce a smooth-walled preparation with no dentine overhangs
- prevent damage to the floor of the pulp chamber

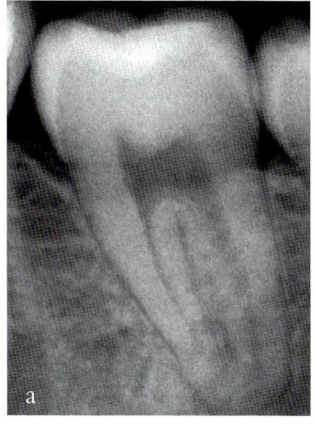

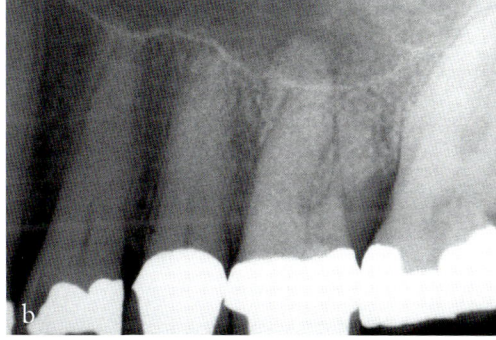

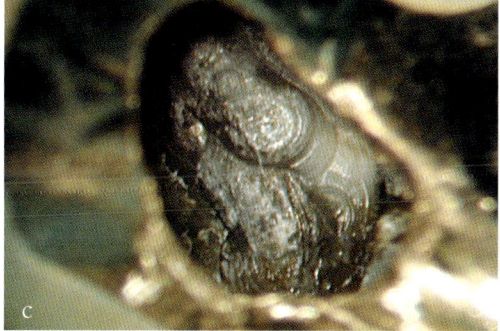

Fig 1-8 (a) Full exposure of the pulp chamber and patent canals should result in uncomplicated negotiation and preparation. (b) The pulp chamber and canals of the upper left first permanent molar appear to be completely sclerosed. (c) Removal of the crown may improve the likelihood of identifying canal entrances.

- allow straight-line access of instruments into the main root canals
- preserve as much sound coronal tooth tissue as possible within the constraints presented by the other objectives (Fig 1-9).

Instrumentation and disinfection of the root canal space
The aims of this stage of endodontic treatment are to:
- debride and disinfect the root canal space
- prepare a suitable root canal shape for subsequent three-dimensional sealing (obturation) with root filling material
- preserve as much structurally important tooth tissue as possible, consistent with the other factors.

Micro-organisms exist both within the main root canal space and in a biofilm coating the complex ramifications of the root canal. The operator can rarely see, let alone enter and fully debride the root canal space with instruments (Fig 1-10). Instrumentation (*debridement*) removes material from some areas of the root canal wall and opens up the pulp space with its ramifications for deep exchange of antimicrobial irrigants and medicaments (*disinfection*). Instrumentation should create a root canal which is three-dimensionally tapered from apex to coronal entrance, and follows closely the outline of the root surface. This taper will facilitate the eventual sealing (*obturation*) of the root canal space.

Root canals should be prepared using a crown-down approach, enlarging first the coronal-third, then the mid-third, and finally the apical-third. Regardless of whether stainless steel or nickel-titanium instruments are employed, this approach works sequentially using larger to smaller instruments as apical progress is made; each successively smaller instrument

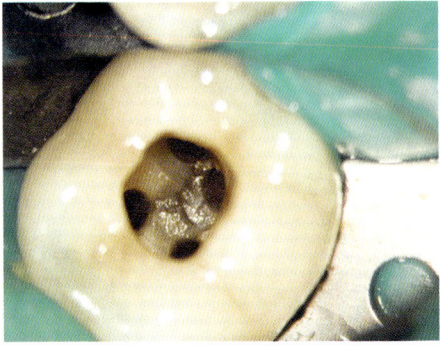

Fig 1-9 Minimally prepared access.

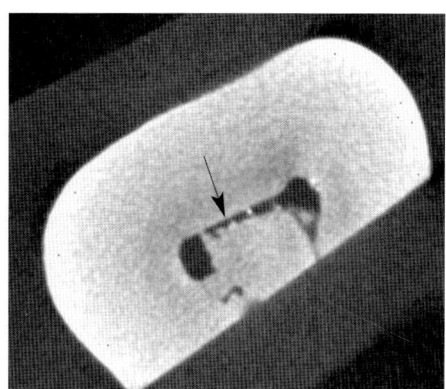

Fig 1-10 Complex anatomy of the isthmus (indicated by arrow) of the mesial root of a mandibular molar as it appears in a microcomputer tomographic image.

advancing slightly deeper than the previous one. This crown–down approach has several advantages over the more traditional "stepback" approach, including:

- Removal of the bulk of the coronal infected necrotic pulp tissue and dentine, preventing its movement apically into the periapical tissues.
- Elimination of coronal interferences, thus minimising the creation of blockages apically.
- Earlier deep exchange of irrigants.
- Maintenance of working length during subsequent preparation.
- Improved tactile feedback during hand instrumentation, in particular at the delicate root-end.

Mechanical instrumentation can be carried out with a variety of instruments and files systems. These may be manufactured from stainless steel (e.g. Gates-Glidden drills, Hedstroem and flexible K files) or from nickel-titanium alloy (e.g. hand and rotary files of increased taper, such as ProTaper® and Files of Greater Taper®). Straight root canals may be relatively easy to prepare once the working length has been determined. However, canal transportation (e.g. ledging and perforation) can be a problem when curved root canals are instrumented with stainless steel files. Although small sited stainless steel files (sizes 06 to 20) are flexible, larger files sizes are increasingly inflexible and may result in uneven removal of dentine from the root canal walls as a result of the instrument straightening within the curved canal (Fig 1-11).

To overcome these problems, when preparing root canals manually with stainless steel instruments, rotational techniques, such as "balance-force"

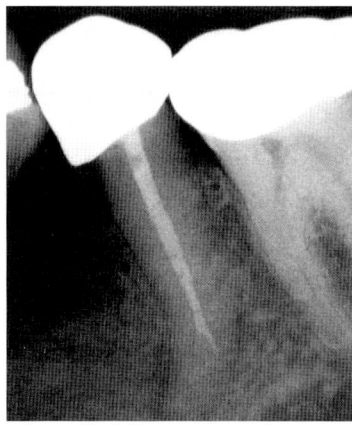

Fig 1-11 Premature instrumentation with large, inflexible stainless steel files has resulted in deviation from the long axis of the canal, with apical third ledging and blockage. The prognosis will be compromised if the obstruction cannot be bypassed.

motion should be employed, ideally with instruments carrying modified non-end cutting tips to enhance instrument centring and reducing the risk of gouging canal walls.

The introduction of hand and rotary nickel-titanium files in the 1990s revolutionised root canal instrumentation. Nickel-titanium files have shape memory and super-elastic characteristics. Shape memory allows the file to return to its original shape after it has been used; super-elasticity means that the files retain their flexibility with increased diameters compared to the equivalent sized stainless steel files (Fig 1-12a,b). Nickel-titanium files also have an increased resistance to torsional failure, thus allowing them to be used more safely in rotary motion within curved root canals. These instruments are machined with innovative design features (e.g. non-cutting tips, increased tapers, radial lands) resulting in well-centred canal preparations and significantly less canal aberrations in curved root canals compared to stainless steel instruments. Care must be taken when using rotary nickel-titanium files, given their relatively aggressive cutting action and large tapers which can result in over-preparation of the root canal.

Ideally, canal preparation should terminate at the apical constriction, the narrowest point of the root canal. The use of an electronic apex locator in conjunction with radiographs is the most accurate method of identifying the position of the apical foramen, from which the apical constriction can be calculated. Generally, electronic apex locators are good at determining when a file reaches the periodontal ligament (the apical foramen). This is described,

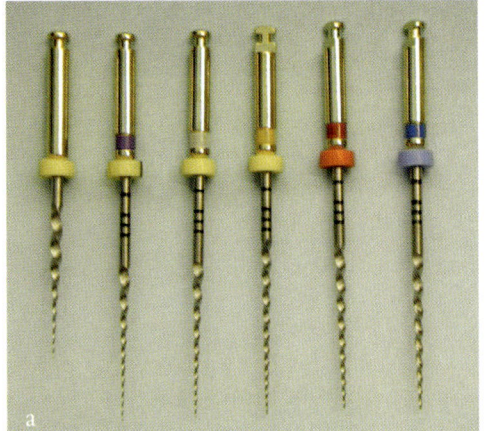 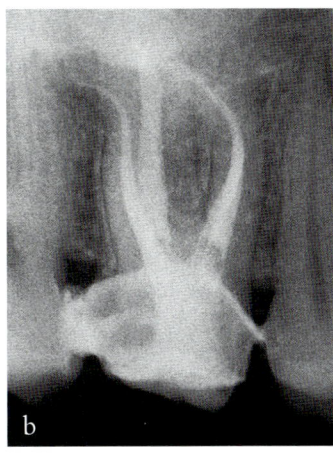

Fig 1-12 (a) ProTaper® nickel-titanium files, the taper varies along the shank of each instrument. (b) Severely curved root canals in the upper right first permanent molar have been prepared using a combination of stainless steel and nickel-titanium instruments. The original curvatures of the canal have been maintained.

normally, as a "zero reading", from which 0.5–1.0 mm is usually subtracted to determine the working length within the tooth (the apical constriction). Once the working length has been determined, the apical third of the root canal can be prepared using stainless steel and nickel-titanium files.

The final shape (taper) of the root canal preparation should be determined by the unique root canal anatomy of the tooth being treated, not by the dictat of file manufacturers and file designs. Moreover, this will help in maintaining sound tooth structure which will be essential in improving the life expectancy of the tooth (Fig 1-13a,b).

At present, sodium hypochlorite is considered the most suitable root canal irrigant, combining general features of instrument lubrication and flushing of debris with antimicrobial and collagen-dissolving activity. The root canal irrigant should be replenished regularly since the active free chlorine ions are rapidly depleted, the irrigant should be agitated regularly to allow it to circulate into the more inaccessible areas of the root canal space. Ethylenediamine tetra-acetic acid (EDTA) may enhance the disinfection of the root canal space by removing the smear layer and, thereby, facilitating penetration of dentinal tubules by disinfectants. Each root canal should be copiously irrigated for at least 30 minutes prior to dressing or definitive obturation (Fig 1-13c).

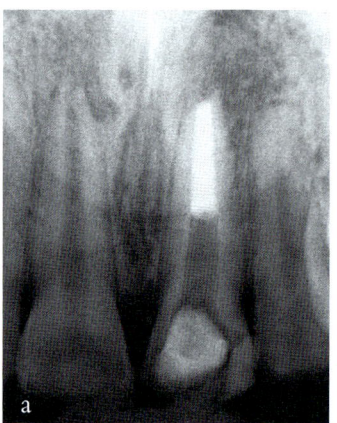 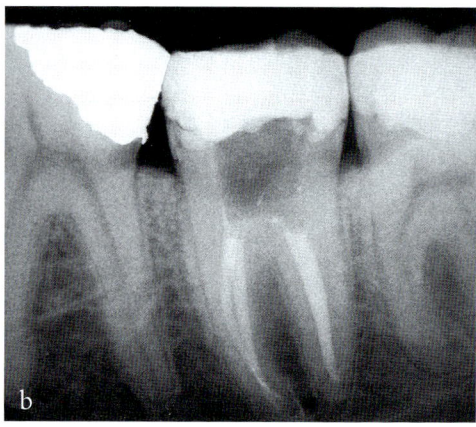

Fig 1-13 (a) This root canal required minimal instrumentation as it was sufficiently wide to allow adequate disinfection of the entire root canal space, and had a natural taper to facilitate subsequent obturation.

Fig 1-13 (b) The root canals of the lower right first permanent molar have been instrumented to allow irrigant exchange apically. Note the significant bulk of root wall that has been left after instrumentation.

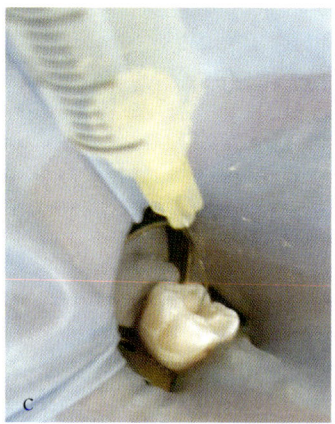

Fig 1-13 (c) Copious irrigation of the root canal space with antimicrobial and tissue-dissolving irrigants is central to endodontic success.

It must be remembered that excessive exposure of dentine to EDTA and NaOCl solutions may have detrimental effects not only on the mechanical strength of the tooth, but also on the efficacy of restorative bonding. These issues will be considered further in Chapter 2.

Root canal treatment may be carried out in a single visit (i.e. preparation and sealing in one appointment) providing there has been sufficient time (30 minutes of irrigant exposure) to disinfect the root canal space after it has been instrumented. If the tooth is to be treated over two or more appointments, an antibacterial medicament such as calcium hydroxide paste should be used to dress the root canal.

Aggressive over-instrumentation of the coronal and mid-third of the root canal must be avoided as this may weaken the tooth, or worse may result in a strip perforation (Fig 1-14a,b). Long-term calcium hydroxide dressing of the root canal should also be avoided as this can increase the elastic modulus of the dentine, thereby increasing the likelihood of root fracture.

Sealing the Root Canal Space
The aims of obturation are to:
- prevent reinfection of the disinfected root canal space by oral micro-organisms
- entomb any remaining micro-organisms within the root canal space
- prevent entry of periapical tissue fluid into the root canal space, as it may act as a nutritional supply for any remaining micro-organisms.

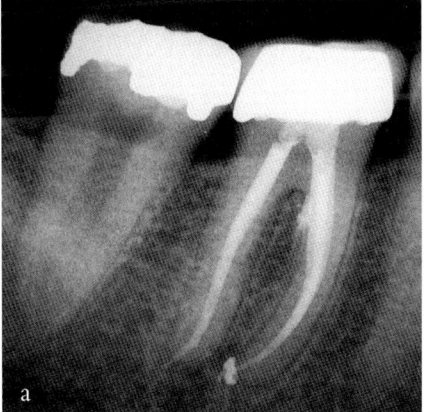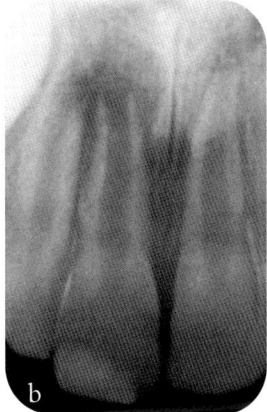

Fig 1-14 (a) Excessive enlargement with nickel titanium rotary instruments has resulted in a strip perforation of the inner aspects of the mesial canals of a lower right first permanent molar. (b) This traumatised upper right central incisor will require no mechanical instrumentation as there is adequate radicular access for irrigation. Further enlargement may compromise the already weak tooth, and care should be exercised in compacting the root canal filling if inadvertent fracture is to be avoided.

Lateral condensation is a simple, inexpensive and predictable obturation technique, widely taught in dental schools worldwide. Although this technique may seal the main canal, it does not lend itself well to complex canal systems with fins and irregularities, or to canals with discontinuous taper, such as internal resorptions. Its track record in successful root canal treatments is, however, beyond doubt. To overcome problems of material adaptation and flow, "thermoplasticised" gutta-percha techniques are now in widespread use, resulting in denser and more complete root fillings, even in the presence of complex anatomy (Fig 1-15a).

One commonly used technique (continuous wave of condensation) employs a pre-measured, electrically activated heated plugger to vertically compact the gutta-percha into the apical third of the root canal. The apical taper of the root canal preparation and snug fit of the gutta-percha point provide suitable resistance form to prevent the gutta-percha extruding through the apical foramen. The middle and coronal-thirds of the canal are then "backfilled" with injection-moulded thermoplastic gutta-percha, delivered by a gun system such as Obtura II® (Fig 1-15b).

All root canal pluggers and spreaders should fit the root canal passively; care should be taken to avoid excessive pressure when compacting the root filling to avoid fracturing the root.

The root filling should terminate apically at the end point of preparation (apical constriction). Coronally, the filling should end 1–2 mm below each canal entrance. In situations where there has been periodontal bone loss, the root filling should end 1–2 mm below the crestal bone level, therefore preventing the root filling from becoming exposed to the oral environment via patent dentinal tubules (Fig 1-15c).

If a post-retained restoration is planned, the post-channel should ideally be prepared immediately on completion of the root canal filling.

How Do Endodontically Treated Teeth Differ From Vital Teeth?

Endodontically treated teeth appear to be more susceptible to fracture when compared to teeth with vital pulps (Fig 1-16). This may be due to the cumulative effects of a number of factors, including:
- *Loss of tooth tissue* – teeth that undergo root canal treatment are often heavily restored, with loss of one or both marginal ridges. This, in addition to further tissue loss for endodontic access, leaves posterior teeth at risk of

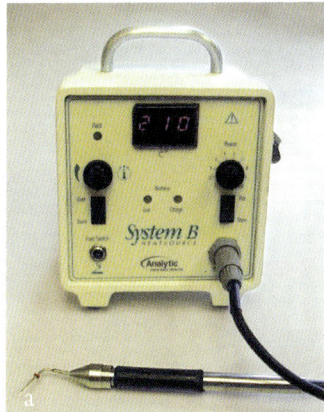

Fig 1-15 (a) System B device for warm vertical compaction.

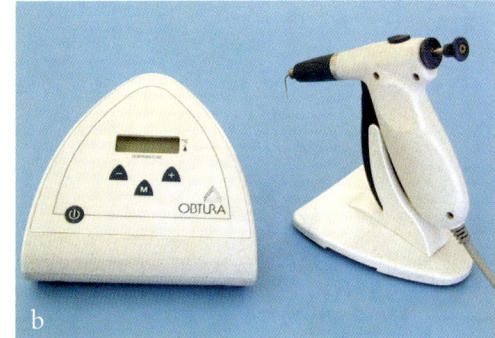

Fig 1-15 (b) Obtura II injection-moulded thermoplastic root filling system.

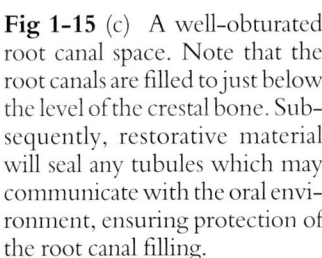

Fig 1-15 (c) A well-obturated root canal space. Note that the root canals are filled to just below the level of the crestal bone. Subsequently, restorative material will seal any tubules which may communicate with the oral environment, ensuring protection of the root canal filling.

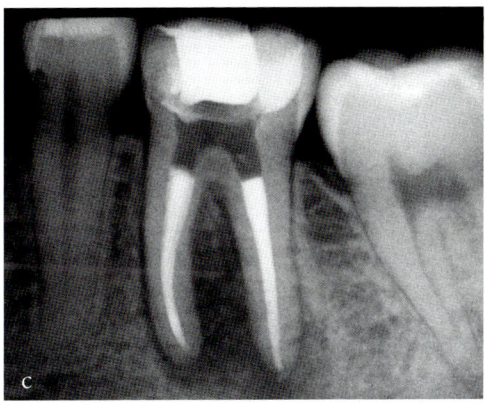

longitudinal fracture under functional loads. Thinning of cusps during endodontic access may also increase the cusp height to width ratio, increasing the susceptibility of individual cusps to fracture.

- *Loss of proprioception* – there is evidence to suggest that proprioceptors exist within the pulp, and that the loading threshold of pulpless teeth is significantly higher than that of teeth with vital pulps. This may result in inadvertent overloading of teeth which already have a compromised volume and distribution of sound coronal tissue.
- *Over-instrumentation* – excessive removal of dentine from the coronal and mid-third of the root canal as a result of over-instrumentation and post-

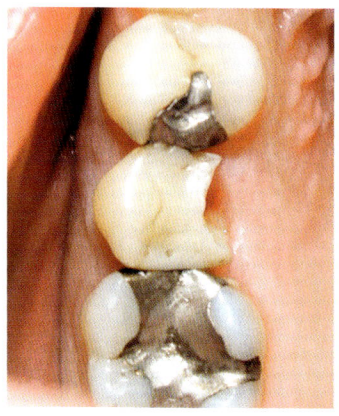

Fig 1-16 The palatal cusp of this root canal treated tooth has fractured 3 mm subgingivally, and the tooth is unrestorable. This may have been prevented by supporting the tooth during treatment and providing a cusp-protecting restoration soon after the root canal treatment was complete.

space preparation may weaken the remaining root canal and predispose to crown/root fracture.

• *Excessive irrigation and/or long-term intracanal dressing* – the excessive use of irrigants (e.g. sodium hypochlorite and EDTA) and/or long-term calcium hydroxide medication may change the chemical composition and physical properties of dentine and promote fracture.

> Again, the root canal treatment should never be considered an end in its own right, and all actions during root canal treatment should be conducted with due consideration to the design and success of the final restoration.

Why and When to Restore the Root Canal Treated Tooth

Once the root canal treatment is complete, the tooth should be restored with the minimum of delay, to:
• provide a fluid- and microbe-tight coronal seal
• protect the tooth from fracture.

Poor quality restorations, or delay in restoration may compromise the outcome of root canal treatment, or result in tooth loss for non-endodontic reasons (Fig 1-17a–c).

If there is sufficient time, and when indicated, a fibre post may be placed and the pulp chamber sealed immediately with a plastic restoration. This is the ideal time to restore, since the access cavity is readily accessible and thoroughly disinfected, and the tooth is still isolated with rubber dam, creating the ideal conditions for restoration. However, in cases where more complex restorations are required, e.g. when a cuspal coverage restoration is planned for a posterior tooth, the tooth may be restored with an adhesive core which may be prepared for a cuspal coverage restoration at a future appointment. When more than one practitioner is involved, effective communication must be in place to ensure that the root canal treated tooth is not left vulnerable to leakage or catastrophic fracture.

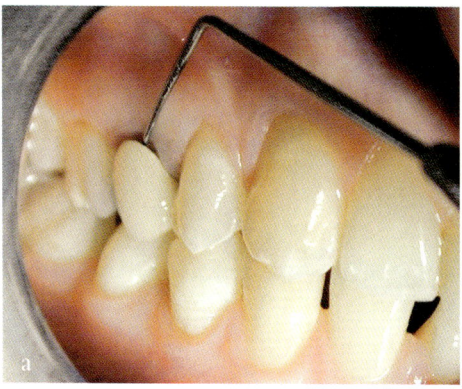

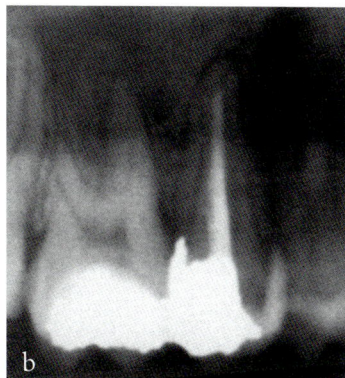

Fig 1-17 (a) Coronal leakage may occur as a result of the poor crown margin.

Fig 1-17 (b) Periapical x-ray taken immediately following root canal treatment, with no evidence of periapical radiolucency.

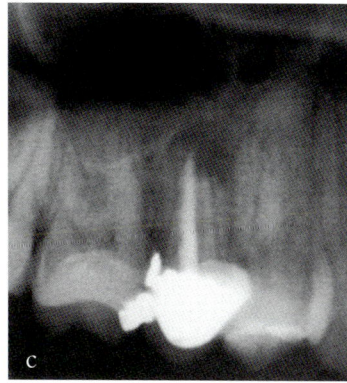

Fig 1-17 (c) A periapical lesion has developed, probably due to coronal microleakage at the defective crown margin.

If the tooth is to be temporised, a layer of Cavit® or a cotton pellet should be placed over the canal entrances and the access cavity sealed with IRM or a glass-ionomer cement (Fig 1-18a,b).

The reported success of well-conducted root canal treatment is in the range of 85-95%. Therefore, provided that the objectives of treatment are met without significant compromise or iatrogenic error, such as perforation, complex extracoronal restorations may be planned one to two weeks after completion of treatment (Fig 1-19a-c). If there are any doubts about the likely outcome of root canal treatment, as a consequence of a persistent sinus or symptoms, the tooth should be securely temporised and complex restorations deferred until there are definite signs of healing. This is important especially in teeth which have been root canal re-treated, where full working length may not have been achieved in one or more canals. In such circumstances, it may be prudent to place a cuspal coverage Nayyar core, or provide a provisional crown to support and seal the tooth before reviewing and making a decision on definitive restoration (see Chapter 3).

The aims of restoring an endodontically treated tooth are similar to those for restoration of any tooth, namely:
- to provide a coronal seal by placing a well-adapted restoration (coronal seal)
- to preserve and protect remaining tooth structure
- to minimise stress within both tooth and restoration.

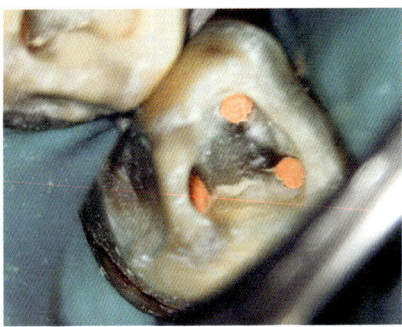

Fig 1-18 (a) A clean access cavity after root canal obturation. Excess root canal sealer and remnants of gutta-percha have been carefully removed to ensure that they do not compromise adhesion of the post-endodontic restoration.

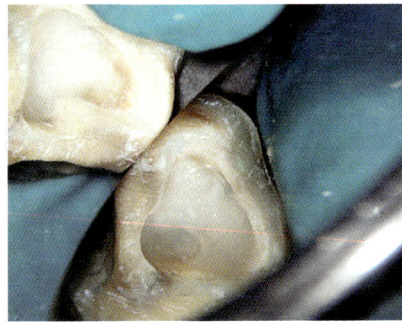

Fig 1-18 (b) A layer of glass-ionomer cement has been used to seal the base of the access cavity.

Fig 1-19 (a) Crown preparation of a root canal treated molar tooth.
(b) and (c) Crown in situ.

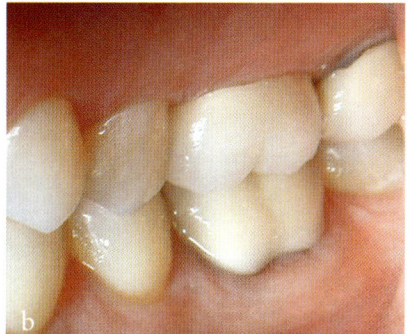

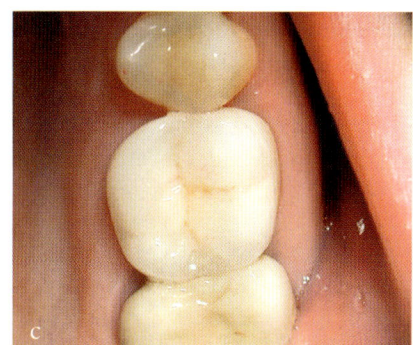

The following chapters will consider the indications for different types of coronal restoration in the rehabilitation of root canal treated teeth, with special emphasis on the role of contemporary adhesive techniques.

When Is Endodontic Retreatment Required?

Root canal treatment is not always successful, studies from many countries having shown that excellent quality work is achieved in less than 50% of cases. Therefore, patients may present with symptoms (e.g. recurrent abscesses, pain on chewing) and/or signs (e.g. tenderness to palpation, sinus, enlarged or new periapical radiolucency) of persistent or recurrent endodontic disease.

Endodontic treatment usually fails as a result of compromised infection control. Specific reasons include:
• Untreated (missed) root canals, due to poor access cavity preparation.

19

- Inadequate canal preparation (i.e. inadequate access for irrigants to reach the working length) and disinfection (i.e. insufficient volume of antibacterial irrigant used), failure to use antimicrobial irrigants (e.g. local anaesthetic solution, saline) and failure to isolate under a rubber dam, resulting in micro-organisms surviving within the root canal space.
- Inadequate sealing of the root canal space and its three-dimensional ramifications, resulting in proliferation or reactivation of existing micro-organisms.
- Inadequate provisional or permanent coronal restoration, resulting in reinfection of the root canal space.

It must, however, be recognised that many root canal treated teeth fail and require removal for non-endodontic reasons, notably unrestorable fracture caused by poorly designed coronal restoration.

The various treatment options (Box 1-2) should be discussed with the patient together with their advantages, disadvantages and prognosis. Only then can the patient make an informed decision on the treatment plan to be followed, i.e. to accept, re-treat, perform surgery or extract. This must be discussed within the context of the overall restorative treatment plan, and the importance of the tooth.

The microbial flora of endodontically treated teeth may differ from that of previously untreated teeth. Micro-organisms such as *Enterococcus faecalis* have been identified in teeth with a failing endodontic treatment. A modified treatment strategy is required to eliminate these virulent micro-organisms, and usually it is recommended in non-allergic patients that sodium hypochlorite is supplemented by an iodine or a chlorhexidine-based irrigant.

Endodontic retreatment should be considered in the following circumstances:
- Signs of failure associated with an inadequate endodontic treatment (Fig 1-20a).

Box 1-2 **Treatment options for a tooth with a failing root canal treatment**

- Treat conservatively and keep under review.
- Non-surgical endodontic retreatment.
- Periapical microsurgery.
- Extraction (and possible replacement with an implant, bridge or denture).

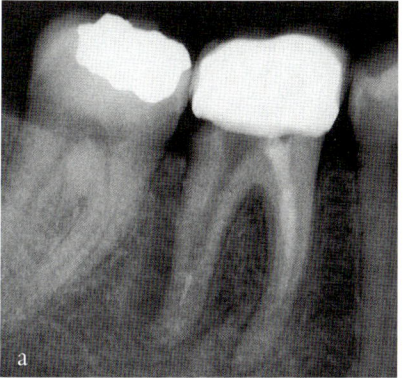
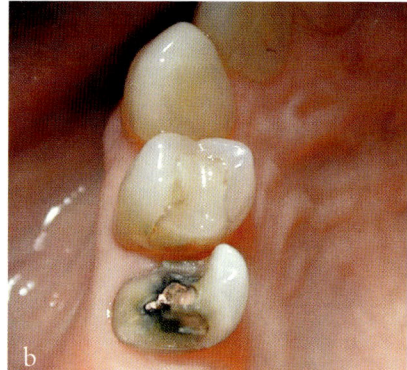
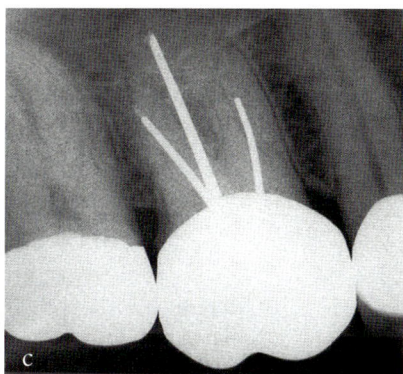

Fig 1-20 (a) Endodontic retreatment is indicated prior to the replacement of this poorly fitting crown. The quality of the initial root canal treatment is inadequate and the tooth is symptomatic. Failure is associated with coronal leakage at the distal aspect of the crown and inadequate root canal treatment. (b) Loss of the buccal cusp and mesio-occlusal-distal restoration has exposed the existing root filling to the oral environment. (c) An inadequate silver-point root filling is scheduled for replacement before replacement of the crown.

- Missing coronal restoration resulting in long-term (more than one month) exposure of a radiographically adequate existing root filling to the oral environment (Fig 1-20b).
- A new restoration is planned on a tooth with an existing technically inadequate root canal treatment (Fig 1-20c).

Rarely, teeth in which root canal treatment has been carried out to a high standard may be associated with signs and symptoms of endodontic failure. In these circumstances, an extraradicular infection, foreign body reaction or cyst may be suspected, for which periapical microsurgery may be a realistic treatment option for tooth preservation (Box 1-3).

When conducted to the highest standards and embracing contemporary techniques and materials, periapical microsurgery may be highly predictable

Box 1-3 **Indications for periapical microsurgery**

- High quality root canal treatment which cannot be improved upon by a non-surgical approach.
- Blocked canal (e.g. separated instrument which cannot be bypassed, sclerosed canal, ledged canal).
- Dismantling the tooth may be damaging or impractical (e.g. long, wide post, post-retained bridge abutment).
- Root fracture suspected.
- Biopsy required.

Box 1-4 **Success rates in endodontic treatment carried out by, or supervised by, specialist endodontist**

- 85% presence of preoperative periapical radiolucency.
- 95% vital, irreversible or non-vital but with no preoperative periapical radiolucency.
- 80% endodontic retreatment.
- 90% periapical microsurgery.

(Box 1-4). However, teeth requiring such treatment may be severely compromised and serious consideration must be given to their long-term survival.

How Successful Is Endodontic Treatment?

The outcome of root canal treatment is dependent on eliminating existing infection and preventing reinfection of the root canal space (Box 1-4). The following factors have a significant impact on the outcome of endodontic treatment in previously untreated teeth:

- *Preoperative status* – the presence of a periapical radiolucency indicates a high bacterial load within the root canal space which may be more difficult to eliminate (Fig 1-21a).
- *Apical level to which the root canal space has been sealed* – an under-filled root canal suggests that the apical portion of the root canal has not been adequately debrided and disinfected. Over-extended root fillings may result in inadvertent extrusion of micro-organisms into the periapical tissues (Fig 1-21b).
- *Radiographic quality of root filling* – voids within the root filling allow micro-organisms to proliferate.

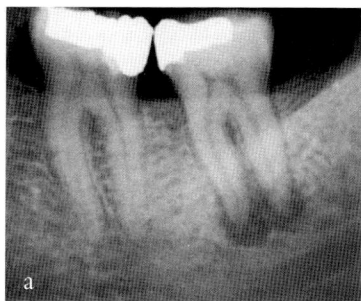

Fig 1-21 (a) The success rate of root canal treatment is approximately 10% lower in teeth with apical periodontitis than in those without apical periodontitis.

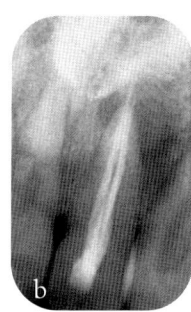

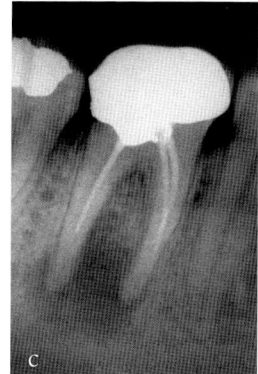

Fig 1-21 (b) Over-extended and porous root fillings are indicators of inadequate root canal treatment. Such teeth may be unpredictable foundations for expensive coronal restorations. (c) Coronal leakage and under-filled (and, therefore, under-prepared) root canals increase the likelihood of endodontic failure.

- *Quality of the coronal seal* – poor quality coronal seal will create an avenue for the ingress of nutrients for any residual micro-organisms in the root canal, and will be a portal for reinfection (Fig 1-21c).

In addition to the above, the prognosis of endodontic retreatment is dependent on being able to completely retrieve the existing root filling material and being able to reach the apical constriction, after which the root canal space can be adequately debrided, disinfected and sealed.

Conclusion

Successful root canal treatment is based on disinfection and prevention of reinfection of the root canal space. Once these objectives have been achieved, the tooth can be restored. In planning and conducting root canal treatment, the clinician should always remember the impact of their decisions, procedures and potential errors on tooth restoration and long-term survival.

Further Reading

Gulabivala K, Patel B, Evans G, Ng Y-L. Effects of mechanical and chemical procedures on root canal surfaces. Endod Topics 2005;10:103–122.

Hommez GM, Coppens CR, De Moor RJ. Periapical health related to the quality of coronal restorations and root fillings. Int Endod J 2002;35:680–689.

Nair PN. Apical periodontitis: a dynamic encounter between root canal infection and host response. Periodontol 2000 1997;13:121–148.

Ricucci D, Grosso A. The compromised tooth: conservative treatment or extraction? Endod Topics 2006;13:108–121.

Rubinstein RA, Kim S. Long-term follow up of cases considered healed one year after apical microsurgery. J Endod 1999;28:378–383.

Sjögren U, Hagglund G, Sundqvist G, Wing K. Factors affecting the long-term results of endodontic treatment. J Endod 1990;16:498–504.

Chapter 2
Adhesion and the Root-filled Tooth

Aim

To address:
- Principles of adhesion to the dentine of root canal treated teeth.
- Mechanical and chemical interferences with adhesion and how to overcome them.
- The properties of the different bonding systems for the restoration of root canal treated teeth.

Outcome

At the end of this chapter, the reader should be able to identify the issues which must be considered for successful adhesive restoration of root canal treated teeth.

Background to Contemporary Adhesive Systems

Based upon the underlying mechanism of action, contemporary adhesive systems can be divided into:
- etch-and-rinse adhesives
- self-etching adhesives
- glass-ionomer systems.

If consideration is given to the number of steps needed to obtain adhesion to dentine, adhesive systems may be classified as three-step, two-step or one-step. Dentine bonding systems will be described according to this classification.

Three-step Systems
Three step systems include:
- Etching dentine with phosphoric acid (32–37%) to remove smear layer, open dentinal tubules and expose collagen fibres on the dentine surface.
- Priming dentine with an hydrophilic solution containing alcohol, water or acetone and resin to establish a preliminary link to the dentinal collagen.

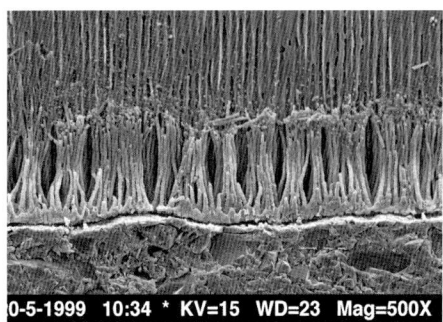

0-5-1999   10:34 * KV=15   WD=23   Mag=500X

Fig 2-1 Intracanal section showing the resin–dentine interdiffusion zone created by a three-step adhesive system.

• Application of an adhesive, methacrylate-based resin that will connect the subsequently applied composite resin to the pre-impregnated dentinal surface (Fig 2-1).

This procedure results in the formation of an acid-resistant, resin-infiltrated collagen layer (hybrid layer) that ensures, together with the penetration of the resin into the dentinal tubules, good bonding of the composite to the dentine.

After the initial etching phase, a 30 s rinse with water is always indicated, followed by gentle air drying of the surface. Complete desiccation of the dentine causes the exposed collagen fibres to collapse, and compromises their ability to interact with the bonding resin. Therefore, the dentine surface should remain moist to ensure that collagen fibres remain in an erect, hydrated state for optimal interaction and adhesion.

Two-step Systems
Two-step systems include:
• A refined version of the three-step system, in which a "one bottle" adhesive consisting of a combined primer and adhesive is applied after tooth preparation and etching.
> Step 1: total etching with phosphoric acid, rinsing with water and gentle drying, as for three-step systems.
> Step 2: application of the combined primer and adhesive.

• Self-etching adhesives
An acidic primer partially dissolves and infiltrates the smear layer and a methacrylic resin that links the primer to the composite resin restorative or luting cement is then applied (Fig 2-2).

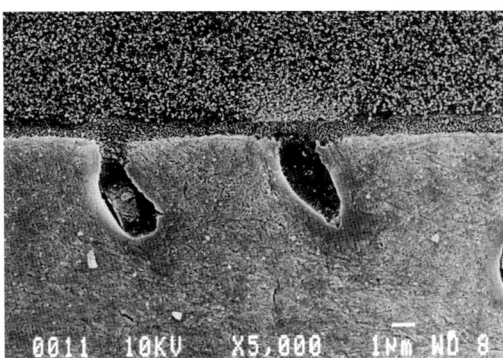

Fig 2-2 The resin–dentine interdiffusion zone created by a self-etching adhesive system.

Step 1: application of a self-etching primer.
Step 2: application of adhesive.

- Glass-ionomer systems.
  Glass-ionomer cements bond to dentine by mechanical and chemical means. Dentine is usually pretreated with polyalkenoic acid to remove the smear layer and expose collagen fibrils to a depth of 0.5–1.0 µm. Interdiffusion with components of the glass–ionomer cement develops micromechanical adhesion by the principle of hybridisation. In addition, chemical bonding is obtained by ionic interaction of the carboxyl groups of the polyalkenoic acid with calcium ions of the hydroxyapatite which remained attached to the collagen fibrils. This additional chemical adhesion may be beneficial in terms of resistance to hydrolytic degradation. Consequently, a two-fold bonding mechanism is established, similar to that mentioned above for mild self-etch adhesives. The basic difference with the resin-based self-etch approach is that glass ionomers are self-etching through the use of a relatively high-molecular-weight (from 8000 to 15,000) polycarboxyl-base polymer. This limits their infiltration capacity, so that the hybrid layers formed are thinner than those created by the other adhesive types.

One-step Systems
- An innovation in which etchant, primer and adhesive are contained in a single solution.

Anatomical Considerations in Adhesion to Root Canal Dentine

Compared with coronal tissue, root canal dentine contains fewer dentinal tubules and, therefore, the potential for micromechanical bonding is reduced.

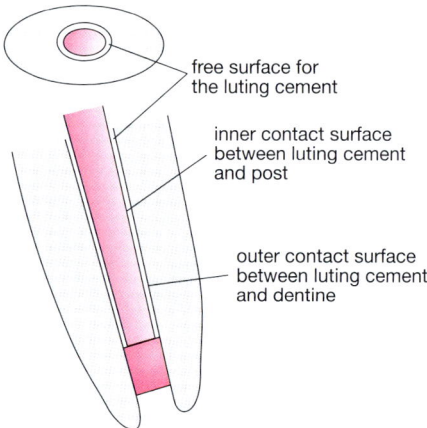

free surface for
the luting cement

inner contact surface
between luting cement
and post

outer contact surface
between luting cement
and dentine

Fig 2-3 Schematic drawing to illustrate the unfavourable C factor within the root canal. The small free surface area leads to high contraction forces within the body of the canal.

Within the confines of a cavity, polymerisation shrinkage can stress or even break adhesive bonds with the cavity walls. The potential impact is modulated by the configuration of the cavity and, as a consequence, the area of the restoration surface, which is bound by the cavity, is free to deform. This ratio is defined as the "configuration" or "C factor". This factor is least favourable in cavities in which the majority of the restoration surface is bound by the cavity, with little free surface to compensate for polymerisation shrinkage. The root canal space, and post-channel preparations, present extreme circumstances in which, depending on the depth and width of the channel, the unbound material at the canal orifice can represent an area some 100 to 1000 times less than that of the restoration–cavity wall interface. Several studies have demonstrated highly unfavourable C factors and predict unreliable bonding of adhesive materials to root canals compared with other, more open restorative sites (Fig 2-3).

Potential Interferences with Dentine Bonding Caused by Endodontic Materials

Materials employed at different stages of root canal treatment have the ability to compromise adhesion between bonding systems and dentine. Examples include:

• sodium hypochlorite
• chelating agents such as EDTA

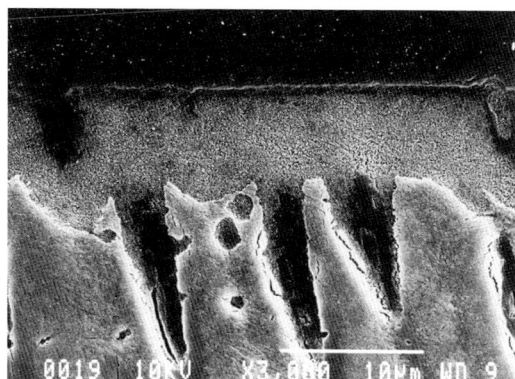

Fig 2-4 Interface between 5% sodium hypochlorite-treated dentine and an adhesive system. Note the wide resin–dentine interdiffusion zone.

- calcium hydroxide
- endodontic sealers
- gutta-percha.

Sodium Hypochlorite

Sodium hypochlorite remains the current "gold standard" for root canal irrigation (see Chapter 1), but its use is not without risks. Concerns have been expressed that the collagen-dissolving effects of sodium hypochlorite may reduce the quantity of collagen present on root canal walls for bonding. Bond strength studies have presented conflicting data, but the majority have reported an increase in bond strengths after dentine exposure to sodium hypochlorite (Fig 2-4).

Chelating Agents

Ethylenediamine tetra-acetic acid (EDTA) is a chelating agent employed widely in root canal treatment. Sequestration of calcium ions from the dentine surface may ease canal negotiation and enlargement, and promote smear layer removal. But it is also conceivable that alteration of the root canal surface by EDTA may result in depletion of calcium ions, microsoftening and compromised bonding. A number of studies have identified this as a significant issue, in particular, for one-step, "self-etch" bonding systems.

Calcium Hydroxide

Calcium hydroxide $\left(Ca(OH)_2\right)$ has been widely used in endodontics as an intracanal medicament. It is considered to possess many of the properties of an ideal root canal dressing, acting as a physical barrier, preventing root canal rein-

29

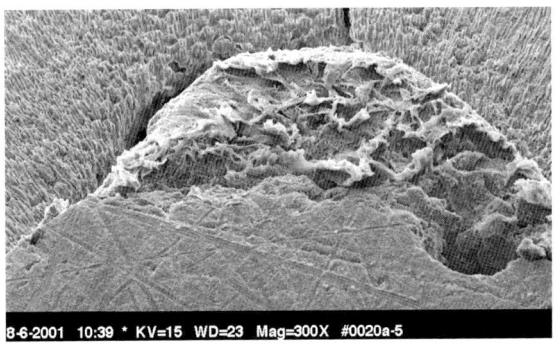

8-6-2001 10:39 * KV=15 WD=23 Mag=300X #0020a-5

Fig 2-5 Absence of resin tags into radicular dentine caused by surface contamination with sealer and gutta-percha remnants.

fection and interrupting the nutrient supply to any residual micro-organisms. The use of $Ca(OH)_2$ in endodontic procedures has been shown to have no detrimental effect on the bond strengths of adhesive resin systems to dentine.

Endodontic Sealers and Gutta-Percha

Endodontic filling materials may interfere with bonding by non-specific and specific mechanisms:

- *Non-specific:* simple smearing of potentially bondable dentine with gutta-percha and/or sealer (Fig 2-5).
- *Specific:* direct chemical interaction between components of endodontic materials (e.g. eugenol) and those of bonding systems.

Smeared materials can be macroscopically removed from tooth tissue with fine ultrasonic tips, operating under copious irrigation and with the help of the operating microscope.

Concerns about eugenol have focused largely on the disruption of initiators in composite resins and impaired polymerisation. Evidence on these deleterious effects is mixed, but some have recommended the flushing of eugenol-containing canals with absolute ethanol to eliminate residual eugenol before adhesive bonding.

In summary, generally the bond strength of composite resin to the dentine of the root canal is found to be lower than that to crown dentine, but sufficient to ensure the retention of resin-bonded restorations in root-filled teeth.

Adhesive Restorations for Root Canal Treated Teeth

Restorative Materials for Root-filled Teeth

Adhesively retained cores can be created with amalgam, glass-ionomer cements and composite resins.

- *Amalgam.* Amalgam is a strong, forgiving material, which is stable in the oral environment and forms an effective marginal seal, in particular, when bonded to the remaining tooth tissues. It has been a popular material for the restoration of compromised, root canal treated posterior teeth. Several studies have compared the clinical success of root canal treated teeth which were restored with direct composite resin and amalgam. From these studies it may be concluded that composite is more effective than amalgam in preventing root fractures.

- *Composite resins.* Composite resins are well-established, restorative materials which rely on adhesive systems for marginal seal. In the long-term, adhesion to dentine may break down irreparably as a result of hydrolysis, thermocycling and clinical function. Flowable composites are considered by some to have an important role to play in core build-up, presenting a modulus of elasticity that is intermediate between the bonding system and the composite core, and therefore serving as a stress absorber. Microhybrid and nanohybrid composites offer adequate strength for core build-ups, although their ultimate strength is, in general, lower than that of amalgam.

- *Glass-ionomer cements.* This group of materials offers a good seal and effective bonding to dentine, but a low level of mechanical strength. They release fluoride, but there is minimal evidence that this is of any clinical significance. Because of their relatively poor mechanical properties, glass ionomers cannot be recommended as core build-up materials. Their use should be limited to the filling of minor undercuts when teeth are prepared for indirect composite or ceramic restorations and for placement in the deepest part of a cavity as a stress absorber.

Build-up of an Adhesive Composite Core Without Using a Post

The adhesive restoration of root canal treated teeth, and in particular that of multi-rooted teeth is often accomplished without the need for a post. The large surface area of the pulp chamber offers a readily accessible and controlled environment for effective bonding. Natural undercuts are often present to enhance restoration retention (Fig 2-6). Rubber dam isolation is important to ensure moisture control for optimal adhesive bonding.

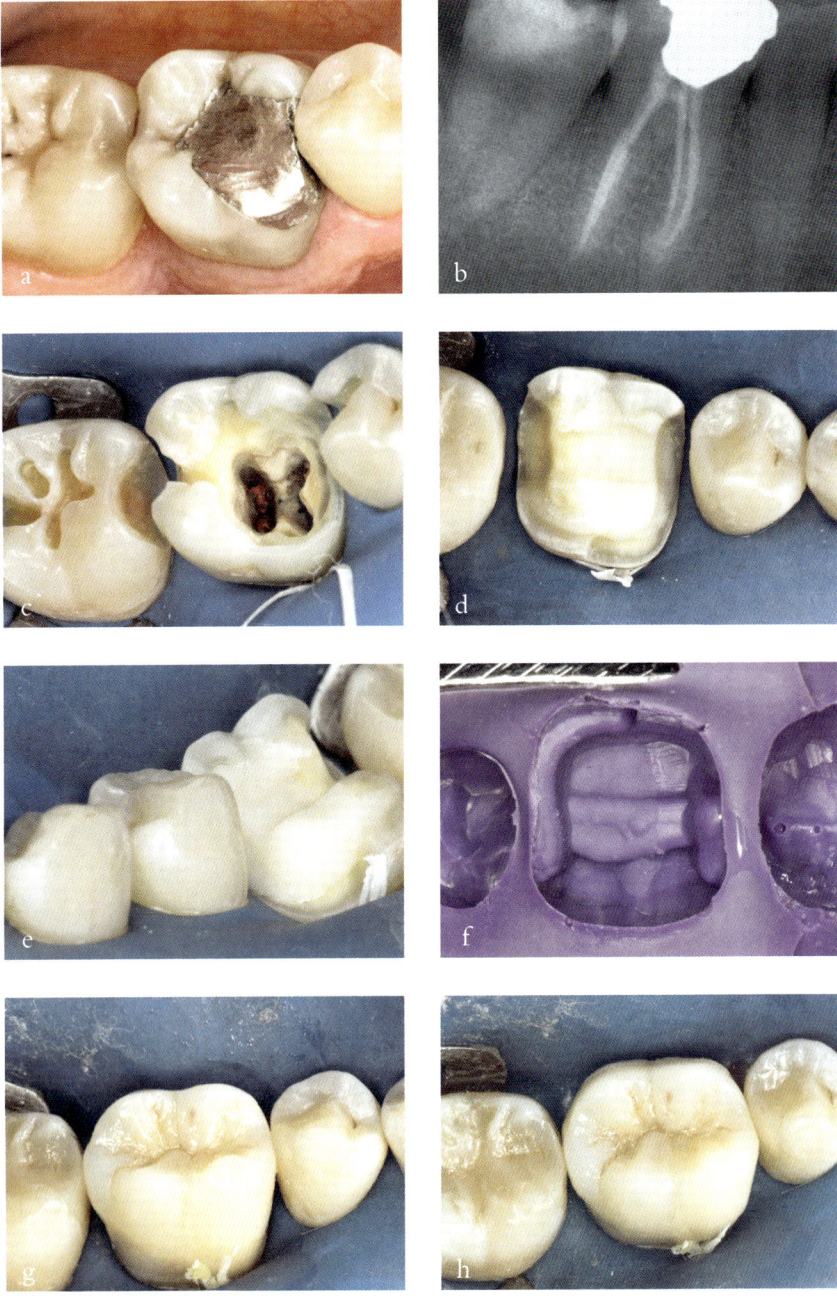

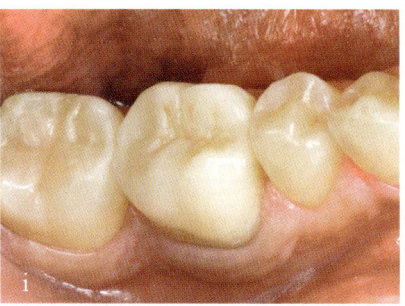
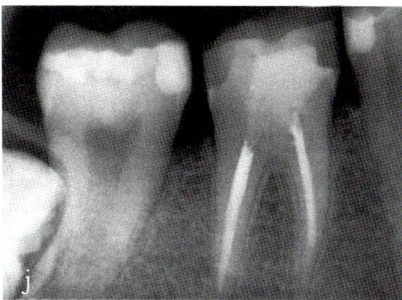

Fig 2-6 (a-j) The lower right first permanent molar was restored by means of a dentine bonding system and a composite core followed by an indirect composite overlay. The residual tooth structure was found to be sufficient to support a composite core without the need of a post. In the review radiograph, the overlay material is not visible given its radiolucency.

Steps required for the direct composite restoration of a root-filled tooth include (Fig 2-6):

- rubber dam isolation
- cleaning of the pulp chamber
- conditioning and hybridisation of the dentinal substrate
- application of a low elastic modulus composite resin or glass ionomer into the deepest part of the cavity, to provide an "elastic" base for the restoration
- application of a microhybrid or nanohybrid composite resin to cover the occlusal surface. The composite has to be applied in increments of a maximum thickness of 2 mm.

Further Reading

Ari H, Erdemir A. Effects of endodontic irrigation solutions on mineral content of root canal dentin using ICP-AES technique. J Endod 2005;31:187–189.

Braga RR, Ferracane JL, Condon J. Polymerization contraction stress in dual-cure cements and its effect on interfacial integrity of bonded inlays. J Dent 2002;30:333–340.

De Munck J, Van Landuyt K, Peumans M, Poitevin A, Lambrechts P, Braem M, et al. A Critical Review of the Durability of Adhesion to Tooth Tissue: Methods and Results. J Dent Res 2005;84:118–132.

Dogan H, Qalt S. Effects of chelating agents and sodium hypochlorite on mineral content of root dentin. J Endod 2001;27:578–580.

Feilzer AJ, De Gee AJ, Davidson CL. Increased wall-to-wall curing contraction in thin bonded resin layers. J Dent Res 1989;68:48–50.

Hayashi M, Takahashi Y, Hirai M, Iwami Y, Imazato S, Ebisu S. Effect of endodontic irrigation on bonding of resin cement to radicular dentin. Eur J Oral Sci 2005;113:70–76.

Ngoh EC, Pashley DH, Loushine RJ, Weller RN, Kimbrough WF. Effects of eugenol on resin bond strengths to root canal dentin. J Endod 2001;27:411–414.

Peters O, Gohring TN, Lutz F. Effect of eugenol-containing sealer on marginal adaptation of dentine-bonded resin fillings. Int Endod J 2000;33:53–59.

Schulze KA, Oliveira SA, Wilson RS, Gansky SA, Marshall GW, Marshall SJ. Effect of hydration variability on hybrid layer properties of a self-etching versus an acid-etching system. Biomaterials 2005;26:1011–1018.

Van Meerbeek B, De Munck J, Yoshida Y, Inoue S, Vargas M, Vijay P, et al. Buonocore memorial lecture: adhesion to enamel and dentin: current status and future challenges. Oper Dent 2003;28:215–235.

Van Meerbeek B, Vargas S, Inoue S, Yoshida Y, Peumans M, Lambrechts P, et al. Adhesives and cements to promote preservation dentistry. Oper Dent 2001;26: S119–S144.

Windley W 3rd, Ritter A, Trope M. The effect of short-term calcium hydroxide treatment on dentin bond strengths to composite resin. Dent Traumatology 2003;19:79–84.

Chapter 3
Crowning Root Canal Treated Teeth

Aim

To review the indications of crowning root-filled teeth, to describe the indications for different crown types and to provide clinical tips on the crowning of root canal treated teeth.

Outcome

At the end of this chapter, the reader should be able to decide whether or not a root canal treated tooth needs to be crowned and to choose the most appropriate type of crown.

Introduction

Decision-making in respect of the restoration of root canal treated teeth is a daily challenge in clinical practice. A variety of restorative approaches have been advocated, most of which can be successful if properly applied.

The decision-making depends on:
- the cost of the restorative procedures
- the risks of tooth fracture
- the aesthetic requirements of the patient
- the success of the root canal treatment or retreatment.

The impact of the cost of the restorative procedures will not be considered in this book. Affordability must always be viewed in the context of the best interests of the patient.

The amount of sound tooth structure remaining after root canal treatment and the amount of tooth structure which is lost during crown preparation are important factors in planning the design of post-endodontic restorations. Existing literature suggests a close relationship between the amount of remaining tooth structure and the fracture resistance of the restored endodontically treated tooth.

It is therefore of paramount importance to preserve as much sound tooth structure as possible. The use of minimal preparation techniques and adhesively retained restorations should be considered whenever possible.

Anterior teeth are less susceptible to fracture and more demanding aesthetically than posterior teeth. As a consequence, the restoration of anterior and posterior teeth will be treated separately.

Anterior Teeth

The life expectancy of a root canal treated anterior tooth is not always increased by preparation and coverage with a crown. Full coronal coverage is indicated:
- if the amount of remaining tooth structure is not sufficient for restoration by direct methods (Fig 3-1a–h)
- when aesthetics are critical
- when anterior teeth are to be used as abutments of bridges.

Restorative Options for Anterior Teeth
Composite filling
Where proximal and incisal tissue loss represents less than one third of the coronal tooth structure, direct composite restoration is usually the method of choice. Bleaching techniques can be used to solve mild discoloration problems.

Ceramic or composite veneer
Ceramic or composite veneers are an option for restoring appearance and function when the extent of tissue loss is less than one third of the coronal structure, the palatal aspect of the tooth is preserved and it is impossible to obtain a good aesthetic result by direct means. Usually, veneers cover the entire labial surface and may extend over the incisal edge and through the proximal contacts. Veneers cannot realistically be extended to incorporate the endodontic access cavity. Partial ceramic or composite crowns are rarely constructed for root-filled anterior teeth as they may be compromised by the technical challenges of incorporating the endodontic access.

Metal-ceramic crowns
Metal-ceramic crowns remain the most commonly prescribed indirect restorations for root canal treated anterior teeth. In order to secure adequate aesthetics a buccal surface reduction of approximately 1.8–2.0 mm must be achieved (Figs 3-2 and 3-3). This may seriously compromise the strength of

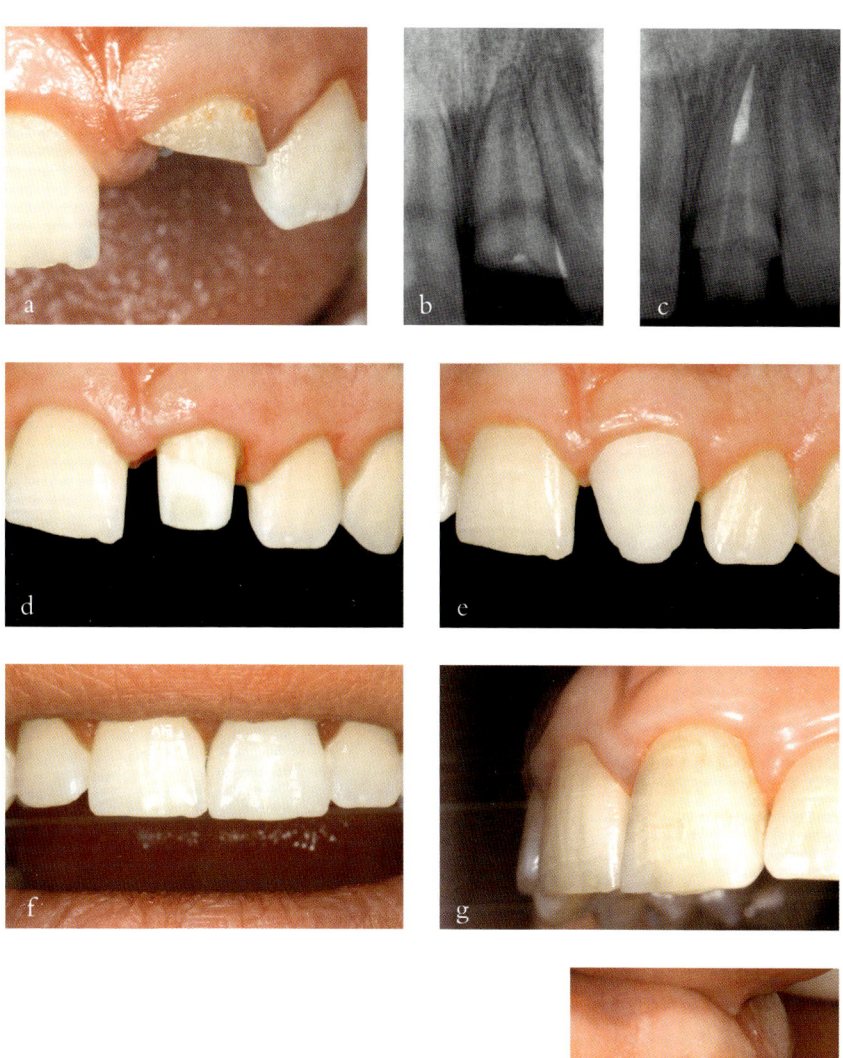

Fig 3-1 (a) and (b) Crown fracture of the upper left central incisor. (c) Root canal treatment and crown build-up. (d) Crown preparation. (e) Ceramic try-in. (f–h) Final result.

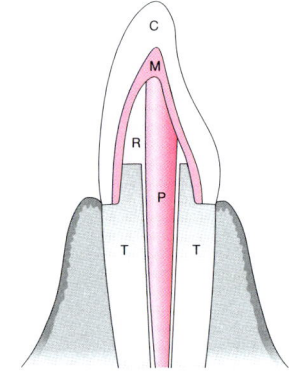

Fig 3-2 Schematic drawing of a tooth restored using a post and a metal-ceramic crown. C, ceramic; M, metal; R, composite core; P, post; T, residual tooth structure.

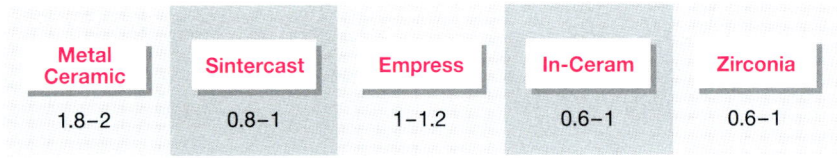

Metal Ceramic	Sintercast	Empress	In-Ceram	Zirconia
1.8–2	0.8–1	1–1.2	0.6–1	0.6–1

Fig 3-3 Thickness required for different crown materials (mm).

any remaining tooth tissue, and caution should be exercised before prescribing restorations, which contrary to supporting the residual tooth tissue may promote its loss.

Captek Auro Galva Crown, Sintercast
These techniques offer two advantages:
• The buccal tooth reduction required (0.8–1 mm) is less than that needed for a metal-ceramic crown, with potential benefits in terms of strength and tooth preservation.
• The colour of the underlying gold allows a better aesthetic result, in particular, in the cervical area. (Fig 3-4).

All-ceramic crowns
Advantages of all-ceramic crowns include:
• More conservative buccal tooth reduction than required for metal-ceramic crowns (Fig 3-5).
• Improved aesthetics, especially in areas close to the soft tissues (Fig 3-1e), resulting from the absence of a metal substructure.

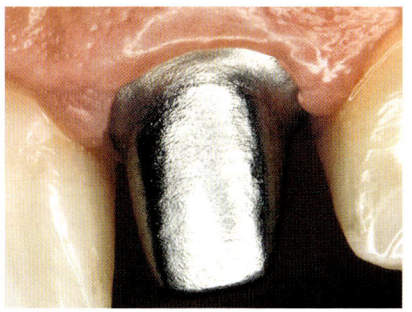
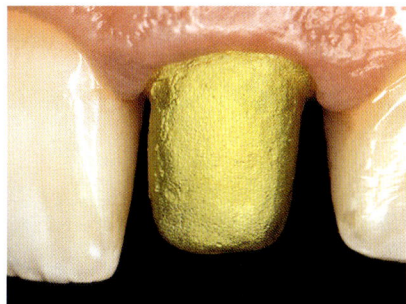

Fig 3-4 The aesthetics of soft tissues is influenced by the colour of the metal used for the core.

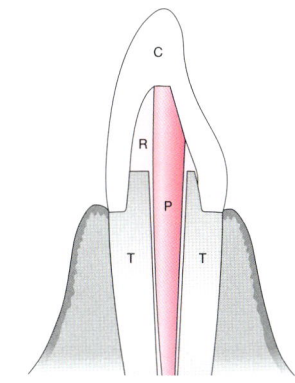

Fig 3-5 Schematic drawing of tooth restored using a post and an all-ceramic restoration. C, ceramic; R, composite core; P, post; T, residual tooth structure.

Endodontically treated teeth are often discromic; therefore, opaque ceramic cores are indicated (Fig 3-6a-f).

All-ceramic crowns are more fragile than metal-ceramic crowns. As abutments for bridges, they are only indicated for three-unit bridges in cases of high aesthetic need. A zirconium construction is indicated in such cases (Fig 3-7).

Gold-resin crowns
Gold-resin crowns have been abandoned due to inadequate aesthetics and the high cost of gold.

Resin crowns
Some authors have suggested the use of all-resin crowns to:

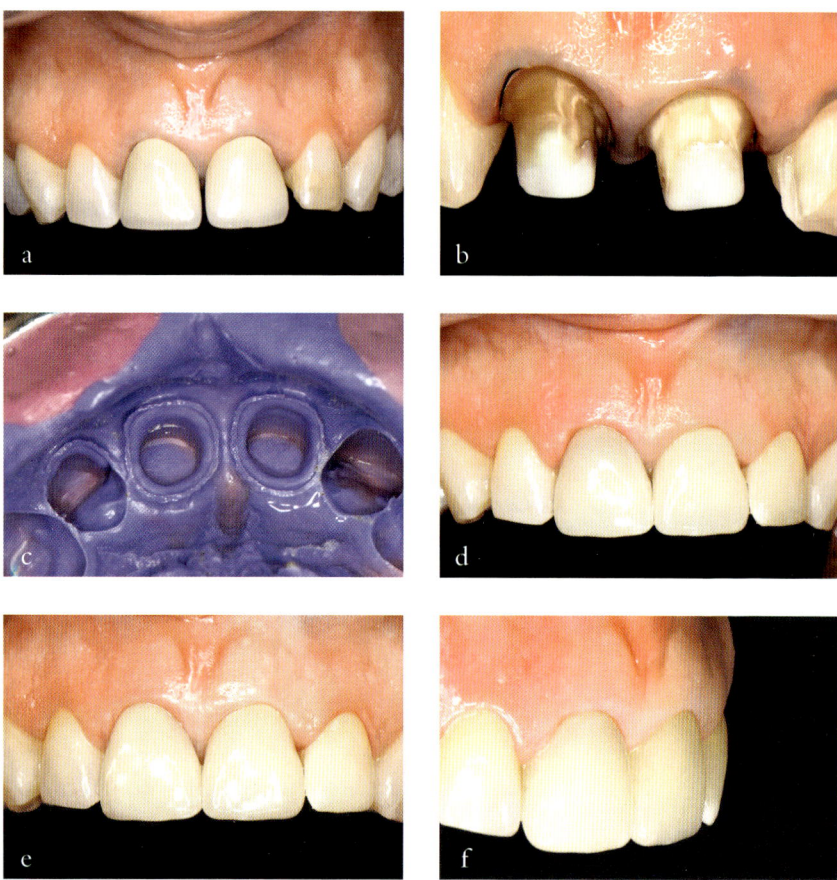

Fig 3-6 (a–f) Improving aesthetics. The crowns on the maxillary central incisors are unsatisfactory because they are too translucent (a). The two central incisors were re-prepared (b,c). New crowns were constructed using a more opaque material (d–f).

- minimise the removal of sound tooth structure (typical reduction 0.8–1 mm)
- allow an optimal aesthetic outcome, in particular, where margins are placed subgingivally
- allow an adhesive cementation.

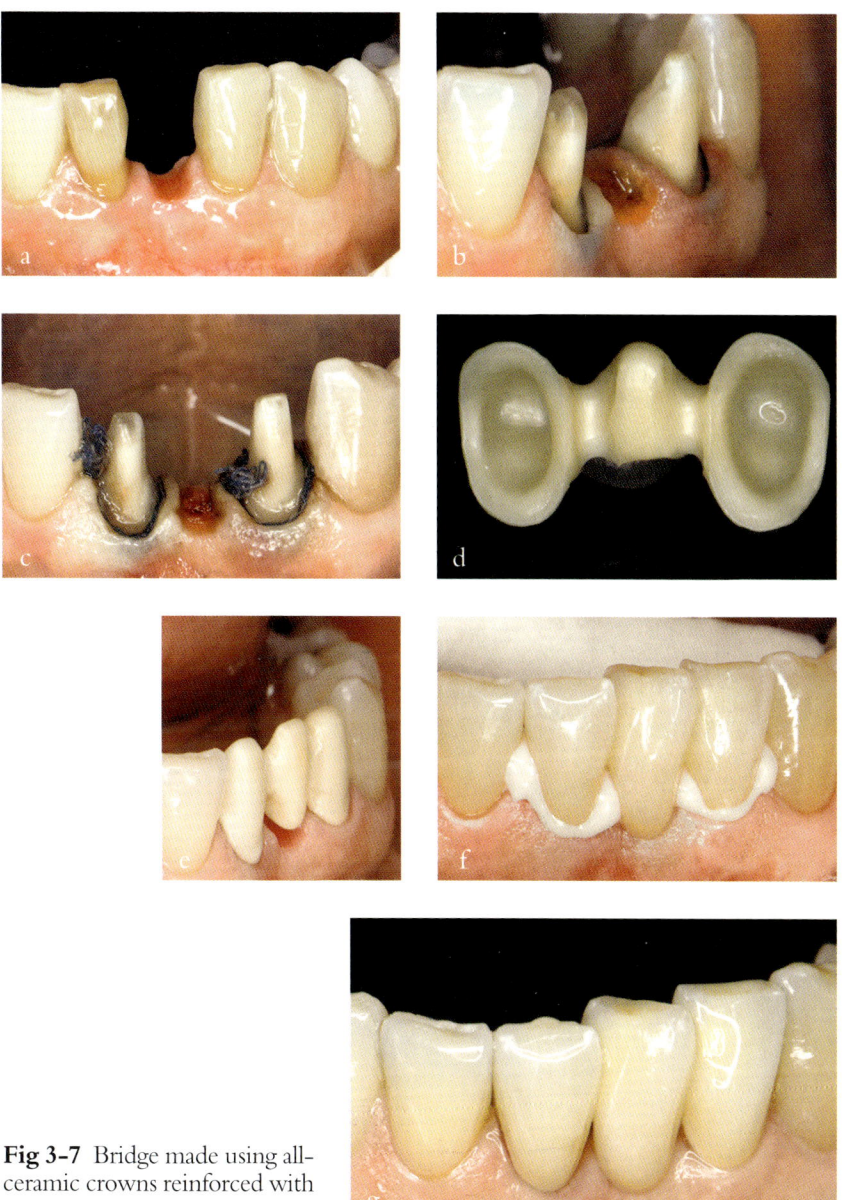

Fig 3-7 Bridge made using all-ceramic crowns reinforced with zirconia.

Unfortunately, resin crowns are just as expensive as metal–ceramic and all-ceramic crowns, but nowhere near as durable.

Posterior Teeth

Endodontically treated posterior teeth are subject to cuspal wedging, high compressive loads and shearing forces, and may, as a consequence, be at high risk of fracture. Cuspal coverage is indicated therefore, especially when one or more marginal ridges are lost. Most clinical studies have concluded that the survival of root canal treated posterior teeth is significantly higher when complete cuspal coverage is provided. Root canal treated teeth crowned as single units survive longer than bridge abutments.

Clinical Choices for Posterior Teeth
Amalgam restoration
- A conventional amalgam, including wide interproximal extension and no cusp coverage is contraindicated, given the acknowledged high risk of cuspal or root fracture.
- Amalgam restorations which provide a minimum of 2 mm cuspal overlay are inexpensive and reliable, in particular in mandibular molars (Fig 3-8), but growing aesthetic concerns have restricted their use in aesthetically important teeth, notably maxillary premolars.
- In maxillary molars, coverage of the functional, palatal cusps is mandatory, while the coverage of buccal cusps may be avoided if they have no contact in lateral excursions.
- In mandibular molars, all cusps should be covered.

If the pulp chamber is less than 4 mm deep, a metal post is needed to ensure retention of the amalgam core; normally a 3 mm extension of the amalgam into the root canal space is sufficient.

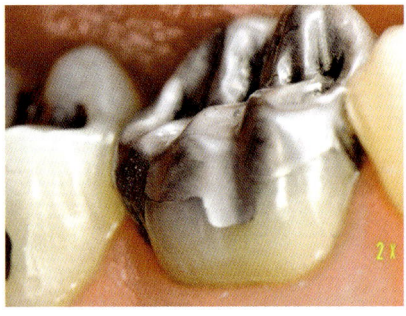

Fig 3-8 Amalgam restoration with complete cusp coverage.

Direct composite
- Many authors consider that bonding restorative materials to dentine may effectively strengthen root canal treated teeth. Unfortunately, it is not yet known how durable the adhesive bond is to the dentine of root canal treated teeth, and whether there is lasting advantage over amalgam.
- There is no consensus on the minimum thickness of direct composite resin required to protect cusps from fracture. Coverage of all cusps with 1.5–2.5 mm thickness of composite has often been suggested. In most cases, direct composite fillings are difficult to perform given the loss of tooth structure caused by caries and access cavity preparation, leaving a large, deep cavity to be filled. Issues may be compounded if cuspal coverage is to be provided.
- In many cases a direct composite filling may result in a poor reconstruction of the coronal anatomy and in deficient contact points incapable of preventing food impaction.
- Composite restorations are regarded as definitive restorations only in cases of limited loss of tooth structure (small interproximal boxes and little or no cuspal overlay).
- In most cases, direct composite restorations should be considered simply as core build-ups prior to crowning.

Gold onlays
Gold onlays are a valuable, durable and conservative option for the protective restoration of root canal treated teeth (Fig 3-9), but have been abandoned by many practitioners given their poor aesthetics.

This type of restoration is still indicated for teeth which are not of aesthetic concern, such as the maxillary second molar. Gold onlays should be offered to patients for whom durability and conservatism are the over-riding concerns.

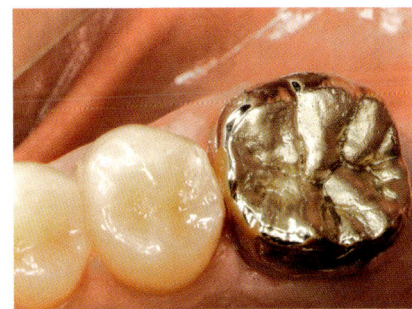

Fig 3-9 Full crown coverage using a gold onlay.

Composite and ceramic onlays

Such restorations are contraindicated in teeth that are to be used as abutments for bridges, are severely discoloured and not aesthetically important.

- Generally, an initial direct, self-curing composite core build-up is indicated, formed by a material which is a shade different from that of the dentine to differentiate restorative material and tooth. This core will then guide the practitioner in designing a preparation for optimal material thickness.
- Normally, posts are not indicated for the retention of a composite core.

The onlay preparation does not differ significantly from that used for vital teeth:

- A minimum thickness of 1.5–2 mm is required for adequate strength of the composite or ceramic onlay.
- Margins should have a 90° finish, and the internal angles of the cavity should be rounded.
- Proximal boxes should only be extended above the contact points.
- Internal walls should be divergent (Fig 3-10).
- Most authors suggest covering all the cusps.

Usually, cementation is performed with resin cements.

There is no clear evidence to favour ceramic or composite onlays, but composite onlays may be less expensive and easier to place and repair.

Metal–ceramic crowns

Metal–ceramic crowns are the most extensively used restorative solution both for single posterior crowns and bridge abutments (Fig 3-11).

All-ceramic crowns

All-ceramic crowns are not frequently used in posterior teeth because of the risk of fracture, although they may find applications in premolars for aesthetic reasons.

Success of the Root Filling

Teeth Without Apical Periodontitis

- If there is tenderness on biting and tenderness to percussion at the time of root canal filling, it is advisable generally to wait two to three weeks before definitive restoration of the tooth. Glass-ionomer cements may be used as a temporary restoration in such cases. If symptoms persist, it may be necessary to repeat the root canal treatment.

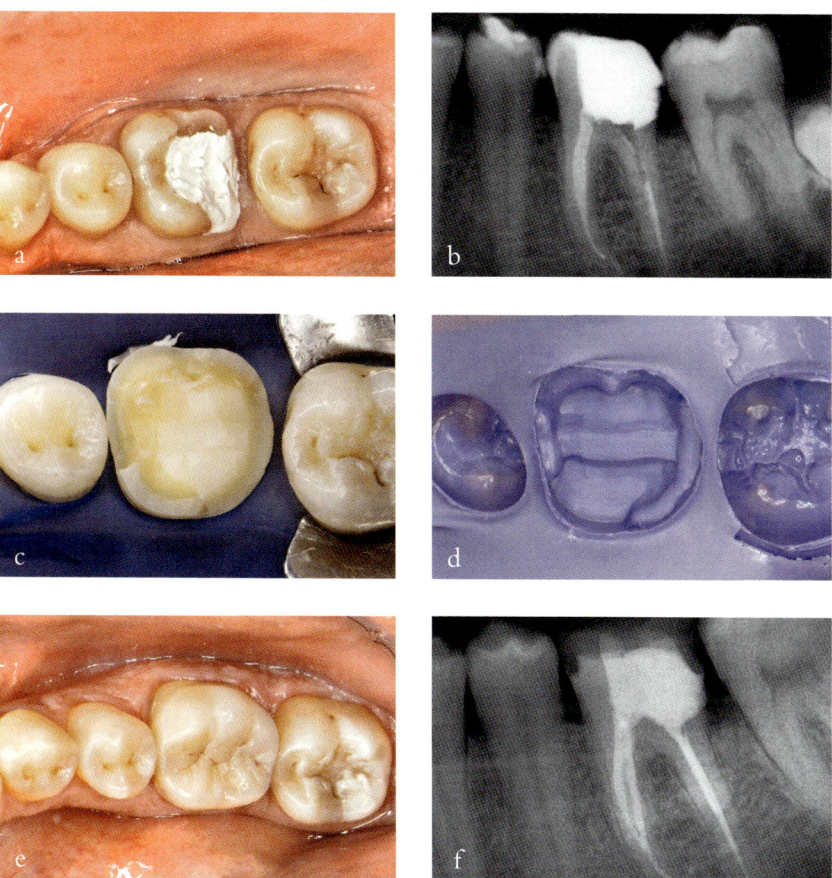

Fig 3-10 (a,b) Tooth 3.6 needs re-restoration. (c) The tooth was re-restored using composite resin. (d) Detail of the impression. (e) Indirect composite onlay is cemented. (f) In the final x-ray the overlay material (Shofu, Japan) is not visible due to its radiolucency.

- If the tooth presents with no tenderness on biting or percussion at the time of root canal filling, restoration of the crown, initially with amalgam or composite, should be performed as soon as possible following the root canal treatment. Composite restorations in anterior teeth and cusp-coverage amalgams in posterior teeth may well be considered long-term (five years) transitional restorations.
- The final restoration (onlay or crown) can then be performed at the convenience of the patient and the clinician.

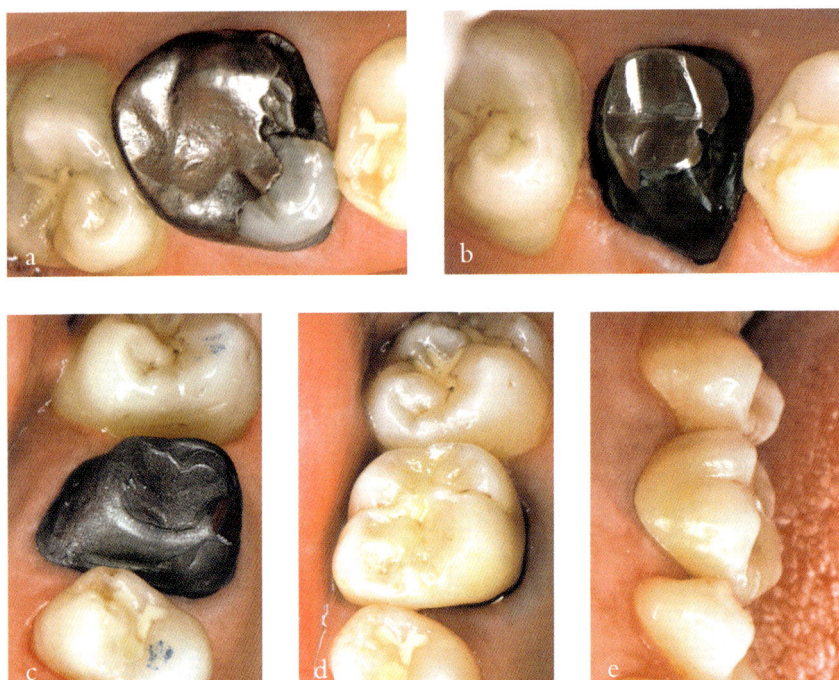

Fig 3-11 Metal–ceramic crown on a root canal treated molar restored using a fibre post.

Teeth With Apical Periodontitis

- If the periapical radiolucency is smaller than 2 mm in diameter, the procedure to be followed is the same as that applied to teeth without apical periodontitis, since the evaluation of the healing of small periapical radiolucencies, especially in the maxilla, is highly subjective. Under such circumstances it is considered reasonable to manage teeth with small lesions in a similar fashion to teeth with no lesions.

- If the lesion is larger than 2 mm in diameter, it is advisable to restore the tooth using a cuspal coverage amalgam or composite restoration, and to review the tooth clinically and radiographically after one year before making a final decision in respect of an extracoronal restoration. If the radiolucency appears to be reduced, the tooth should be restored with a crown or an onlay. If the tooth is to serve as a bridge abutment, a reinforced provisional bridge is indicated for an initial period of twelve months.

Indications for Crowning

Anterior Teeth

Crowning of anterior teeth is indicated only if:

- the loss of tooth structure exceeds one-third of the crown structure
- the tooth has to be used as an abutment for a conventional bridge
- there is a discoloration problem – bleaching must be attempted first
- bleaching is not successful. If the amount of tooth structure loss is limited to less than one-third of the crown structure, a veneer may be indicated.

Posterior Teeth

- Cusp coverage is indicated in all cases in which tissue loss is more extensive than just the access cavity preparation. If the tissue loss is limited to the access cavity preparation, a simple direct composite restoration is indicated.
- Metal-ceramic crowns are the restorations of choice.
- Indirect composite and ceramic restorations may be indicated if the teeth are not to be used as bridge abutments.
- Amalgam cusp coverage is indicated as a transitional restoration; for example, while waiting for the healing of a periapical lesion.

Crown Preparation

In the restoration of a root canal treated tooth, as much sound dentine as possible must be preserved. This can be achieved by the use of dentine bonding, composites and fibre posts (Fig 3-12, and see also Chapter 4).

The term "ferrule effect" indicates a circumferential ring of cast metal or ceramic that embraces a tooth (Fig 3-13) and protects it from fracture.

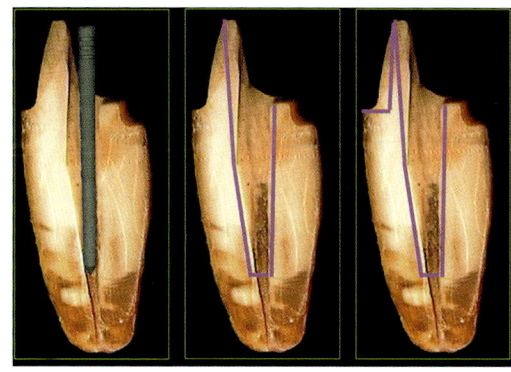

Fig 3-12 A core build-up performed using fibre posts allows (picture on the left) the preservation of more cervical tooth structure, compared to a cast post (pictures on the right). The cervical tooth structure is of great importance in the crown preparation.

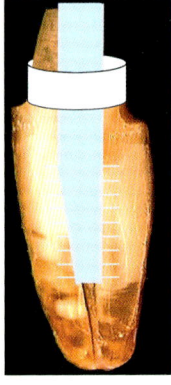

Fig 3-13 Schematic drawing illustrating the ferrule effect.

For effective ferrule protection, a restoration must envelope at least a height of 2 mm of tooth tissue, at least 1 mm thick around the entire circumference of the tooth (Fig 3-14a-c). If the height of the remaining dentine is not sufficient to create an adequate ferrule, crown lengthening or orthodontic extrusion may be indicated (Fig 3-15a-h). In some cases, it may not be possible to obtain a 360° ferrule around the tooth. In these cases, an incomplete ferrule may have to be accepted; providing some support, but acknowledging a degree of compromise.

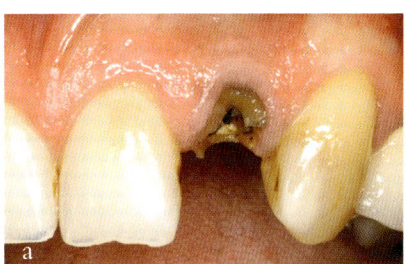

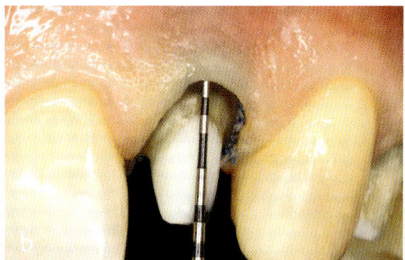

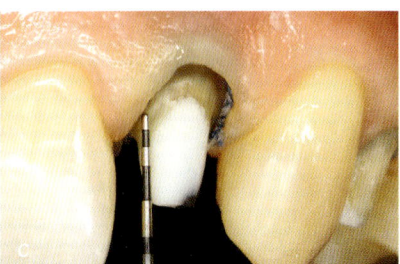

Fig 3-14 (a-c) The ideal ferrule should be at least 2 mm high.

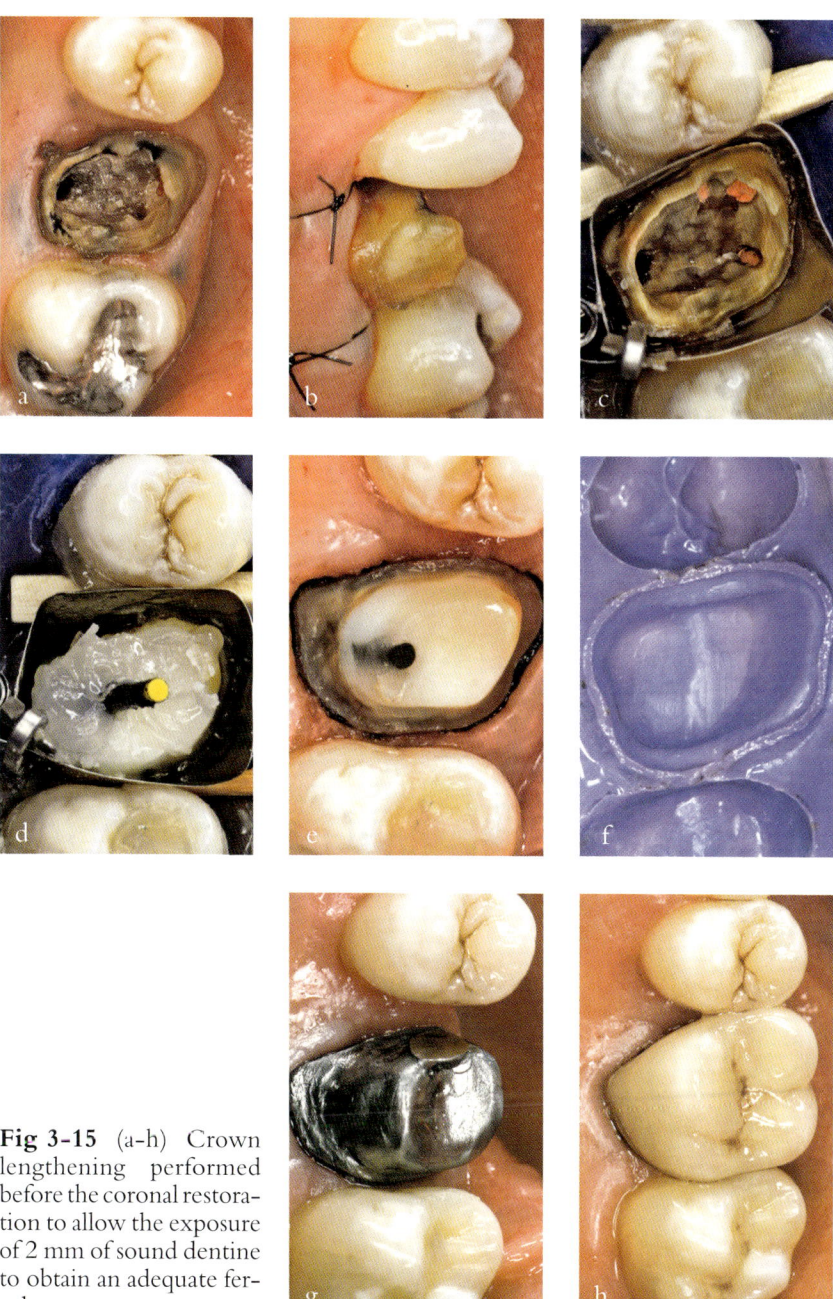

Fig 3-15 (a–h) Crown lengthening performed before the coronal restoration to allow the exposure of 2 mm of sound dentine to obtain an adequate ferrule.

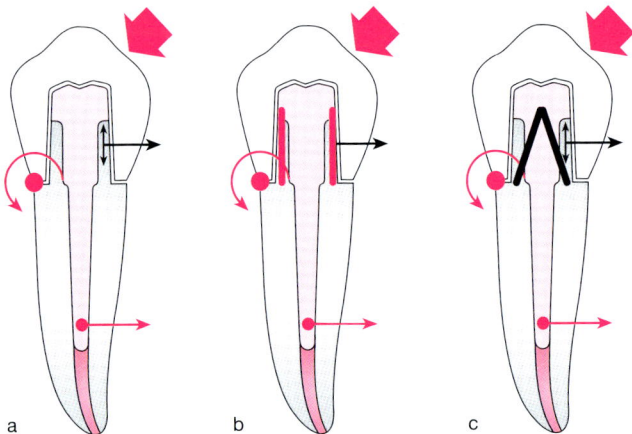

Fig 3-16 (a) The presence of a ferrule around the post increases the resistance to dislodgement of the post. (b) The dentinal walls that are embraced by the ferrule need to be parallel to obtain this effect. (c) Excessive conicity minimises the positive effect of the ferrule and increases the stress applied to the post.

The efficacy of the ferrule effect is strictly related to the conicity of the preparation. The taper of the preparation in the ferrule area must be as close as possible to the ideal 6°. An excessively tapered preparation may result in insufficient retention and resistance to transverse loading. The ferrule may also help in preventing dislodgement of the post (Fig 3-16).

Tooth Reduction
As a rule, a metal-ceramic crown demands tissue reduction of 1.8–2.0 mm to develop acceptable aesthetics and to avoid over-contouring which may compromise the periodontium (Figs 3-2 and 3-3). All-ceramic crowns may demand less reduction (0.8–2.0 mm) (Figs 3-3 to 3-5), but there must be sufficient space to accommodate a stratification of opaque and overlying ceramic to obtain the best possible aesthetic result. The palatal aspects can be prepared more conservatively. A show of metal in the cervical area of metal-ceramic crowns may not be a problem because these areas are rarely visible in normal function. This may be especially relevant for fragile teeth such as mandibular incisors.

Porcelain infusion crowns and all ceramic crowns (Fig 3-17) require less tissue loss and in the interproximal areas a 1 mm wide shoulder may be sufficient to produce a satisfactory aesthetic result (Fig 3-18a-i).

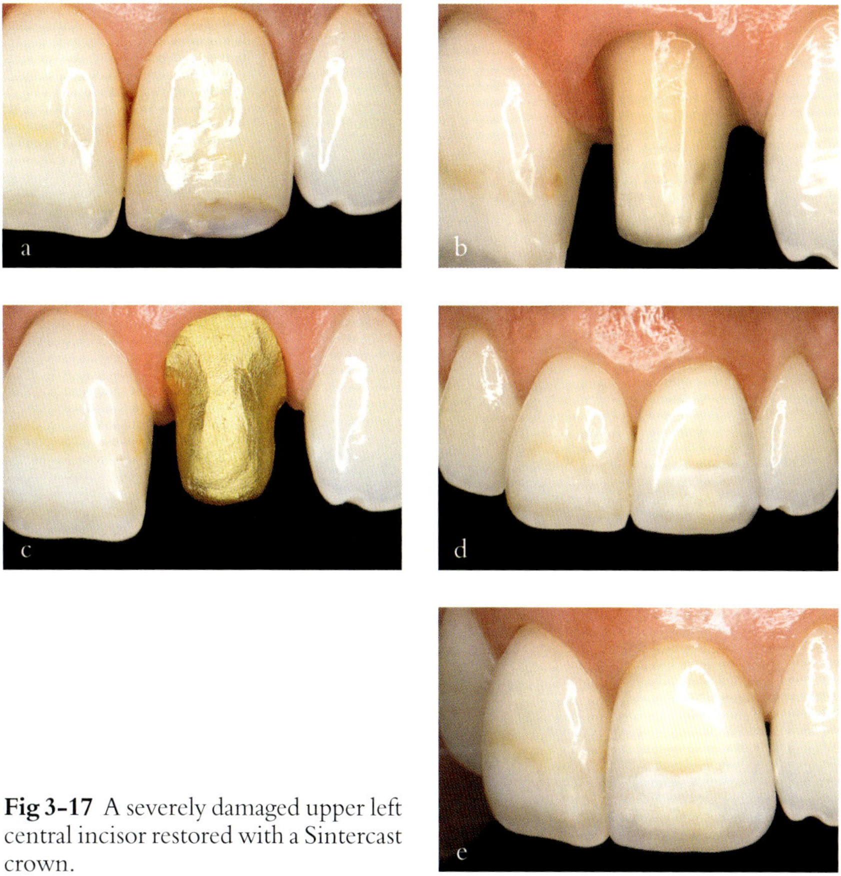

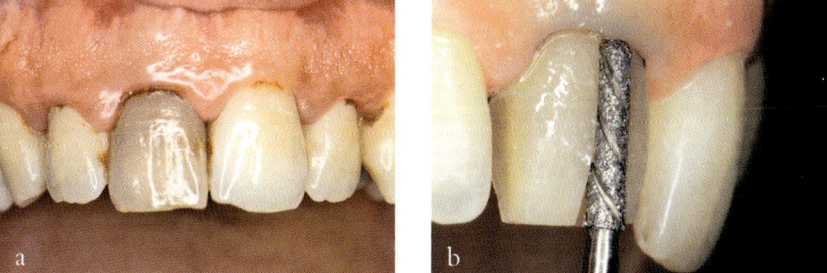

Fig 3-17 A severely damaged upper left central incisor restored with a Sintercast crown.

Fig 3-18 (a,b) An all-ceramic crown is used to restore a severely discoloured tooth (continued over page).

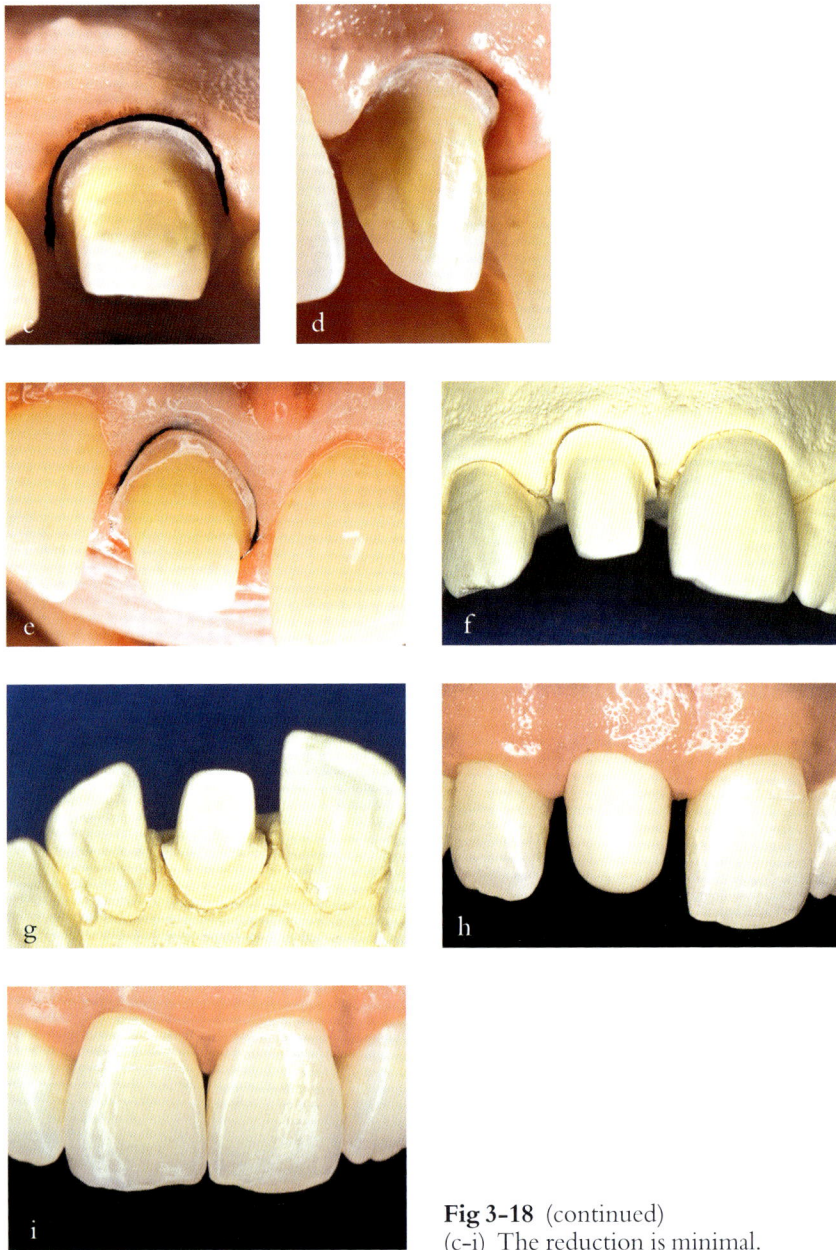

Fig 3-18 (continued)
(c-i) The reduction is minimal.

For the restoration of maxillary incisors, canines and premolars, all-ceramic crowns are indicated because they allow the preservation of sound tooth structure (Figs 3-19 and 3-20). All-ceramic crowns are also indicated in the restoration of teeth with problems of alignment. In such cases, the use of adhesive techniques for the cementation will compensate for the lack of tooth structure available for the crown preparation.

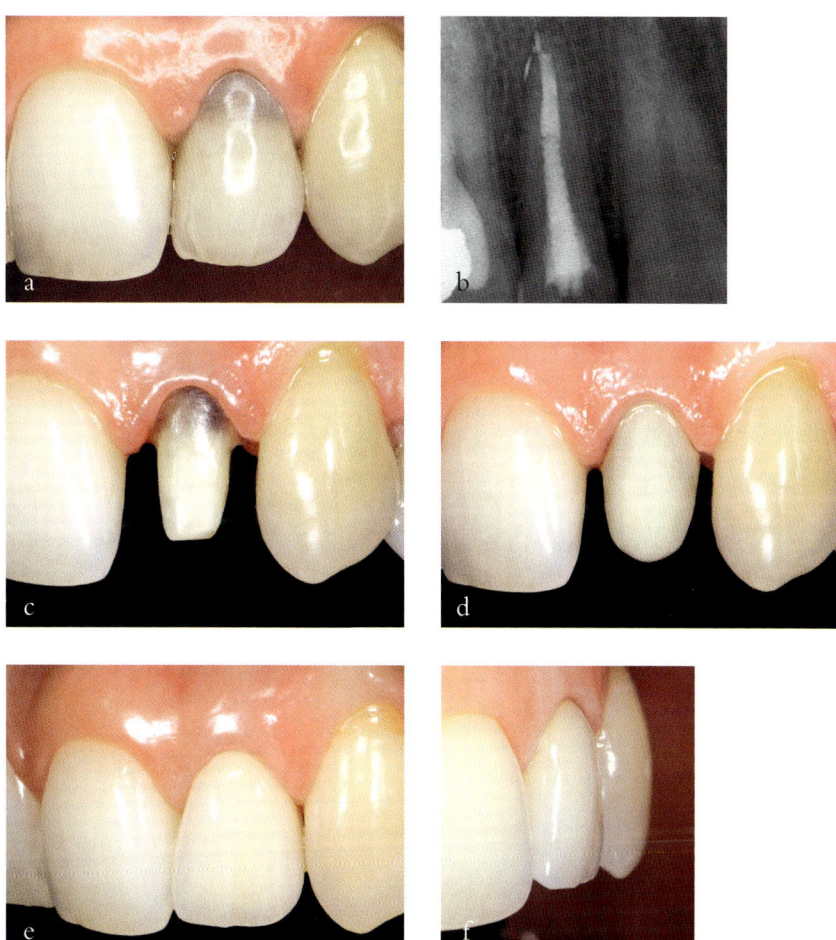

Fig 3-19 An endodontically treated upper left lateral incisor is restored using an all-ceramic crown.

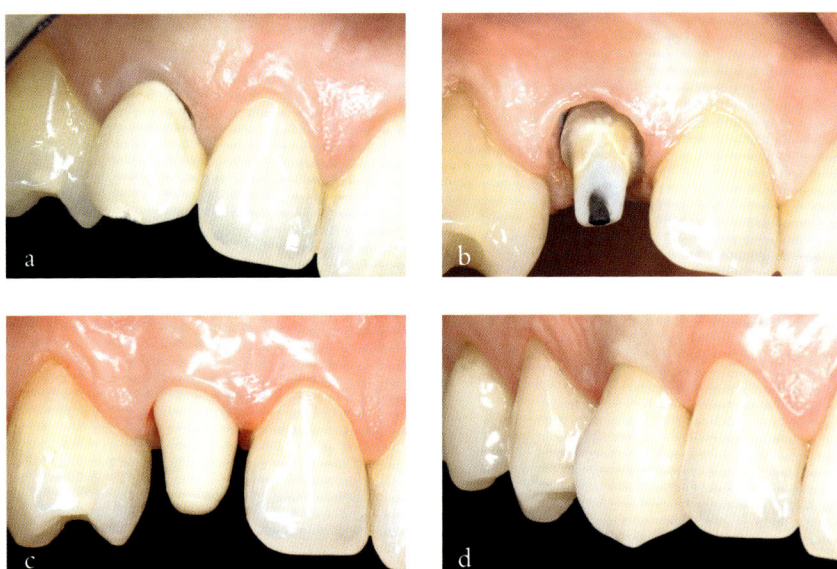

Fig 3-20 A retained deciduous maxillary lateral incisor restored in an adult patient using an all-ceramic crown (In-Ceram Zirconia, Vita, Italy).

Finishing Lines for Single Crowns

A carefully prepared shoulder finishing line allows the preservation of sound tooth structure. The angle between the crown margin and the tooth is normally between 90° and 135°. The width of the shoulder in its buccal aspect must be 1.8–2.0 mm for a metal-ceramic crown and 0.8–1.2 mm for an all-ceramic crown (Fig 3-21). A silicone matrix, made on a diagnostic wax-up, may be used as a guide for the preparation of anterior teeth (Fig 3-22). Occlusally, a clearance of 2.0 mm is required.

A long bevel finishing line may be indicated in posterior teeth affected by periodontal disease. This preparation may be apically extended intraoperatively, involving a periodontal flap.

The Preparation for Bridge Abutments

Bridge abutments need to be parallel to allow the insertion of the bridge. This leads to an increased conicity of the axial walls of the abutments. This may be associated with the removal of most of the remaining sound tooth tissue. For this reason, the placement of a fibre post may be indicated when the tooth is to be used as a bridge abutment. The post and composite core

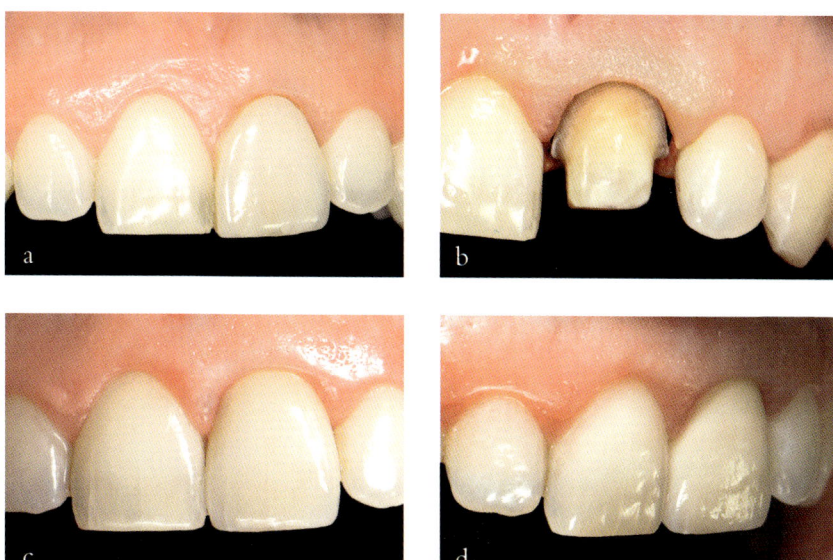

Fig 3-21 Crown preparation showing the different reductions required in different areas of the tooth.

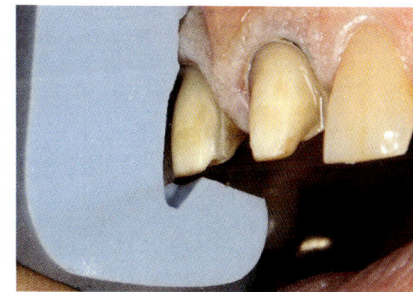

Fig 3-22 A silicone matrix, made on a diagnostic wax-up, is used as a guide for the preparation of anterior teeth.

will provide the structure needed for the abutment. In some cases, the finishing line needs to be configured to facilitate the insertion of the bridge. The creation of a ferrule is particularly important in such cases considering the increased occlusal load on bridge abutments. (Fig 3-23).

Crown Cementation

Traditional cements such as glass ionomers or zinc phosphate are still a valid option. Some types of all-ceramic crowns may be cemented using these

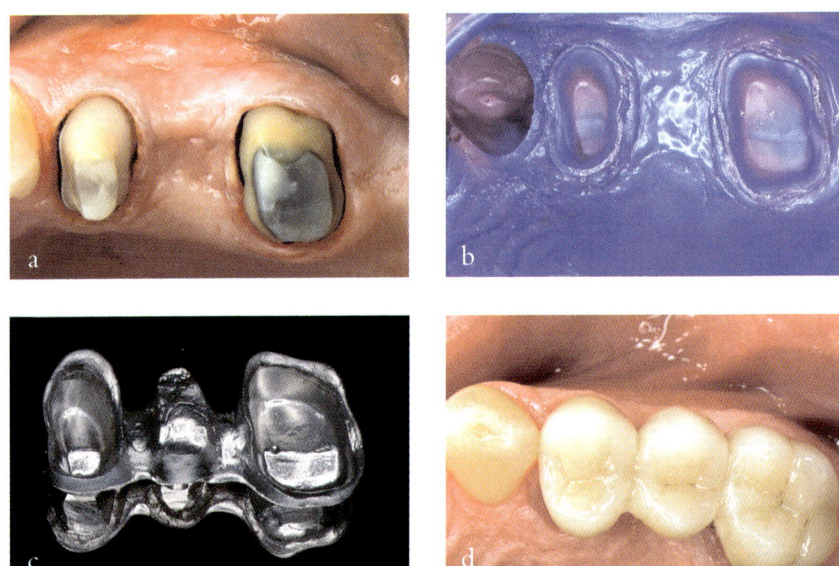

Fig 3-23 Increased conicity of the axial walls of the abutments of a bridge. The finishing line needs to be altered to facilitate the insertion of the bridge.

cements; however, the use of a resin cement (Fig 3-10e) is typical, and a requirement for most types of all-ceramic restoration. A retraction cord may be used to facilitate the removal of excess cement (Fig 3-21b). Cementation using composite cements is more effective if enamel is present at the finishing line. Optimal moisture control is also needed for this type of cementation. A disadvantage of cementation with composite materials is that excess may be extremely difficult to remove.

Further Reading

Cavalli G, Bertani P, Generali P. Finite element stress analysis in post and crown teeth. Giornale Italiano di Endodonzia 1996;3:107–112.

Fugazzotto PA, Parma-Benfenati S. Pre-prosthetic periodontal considerations. Crown length and biological width. Quintessence Int 1984;12:1247–1256.

Gegauff AG. Effect of crown lengthening and ferrule placement on static load failure of cemented cast post-cores and crowns. J Prosthetic Dent 2001;85:96–98.

McLean A. Predictably restoring endodontically treated teeth. J Canadian Dent Assoc 1998;64:782-787.

Shillingburg HT, Jacobi R, Brackett SE. Fundamentals of tooth preparations for cast metal and porcelain restorations. Chicago: Quintessence, 1987.

Stankiewicz NR, Wilson PR. The ferrule effect: a literature review. Int Endod J 2002;35:575–581.

Chapter 4
Fibre Posts

Aim

To describe the types of fibre post which are available and their clinical indications.

Outcome

At the end of this chapter, the reader should be knowledgeable on the properties of fibre posts, and should have sufficient knowledge to be able to cement a fibre post and to build up a composite core.

Introduction

Root canal treated teeth are regarded generally as susceptible to fracture, but the idea of tooth reinforcement by means of the insertion of a post has been heavily criticised. Armed with this knowledge and concerned that post placement may carry other risks such as root perforation, many practitioners have tended to avoid the use of posts wherever possible. If, however, the remaining tooth structure is not sufficient to support a core, the use of a post is the only alternative if a reliable restoration is to be placed, and tooth loss avoided.

The properties of a post-core reconstruction become all the more important as residual tooth structure decreases. Some desirable features of post-core materials include:
- adequate compressive strength to bear functional loading
- a modulus of elasticity to allow some movement in response to functional and parafunctional loading, but without debonding from the tooth or excessive stresses being generated within the restored tooth
- ease of manipulation
- ability to bond to the remaining tooth structure
- resistance to leakage of oral fluids at the core–tooth interface
- thermal coefficient of expansion and contraction similar to tooth structures
- minimal potential for water absorption
- inhibition of dental caries.

Fibre posts were introduced to the market in 1990, with the aim of providing more elastic support to the core, compared to that provided by metal posts. The reduced stress transfer to the tooth structure was claimed to reduce the likelihood of root fracture.

Fibre Posts

The first fibre posts were made from carbon fibres, which were arranged longitudinally and embedded in an epoxy resin matrix. Black carbon fibres were rapidly replaced by more aesthetic white and translucent quartz and glass fibres (Fig 4-1) which are now the standard components of fibre posts.

Mechanical Properties

The mechanical properties of carbon fibre posts were viewed favourably in many laboratory and clinical studies. The performance of quartz and glass-fibre containing posts has led, however, to carbon fibre posts being abandoned.

The flexural strength and the modulus of elasticity of fibre posts were claimed initially to be very close to those of dentine. In fact, fibre posts have a modulus of elasticity that is lower than that of metal posts, but still three to four times higher than that of dentine.

A key difference between fibre and metal posts is that fibre posts lose much of their flexural strength if they are submitted to cyclic loading in a wet environment or to thermocycling. This is related to degradation of the resin matrix in which the fibres are embedded. The failure mode of fibre-post restored teeth is not normally root fracture, as is often the case with metal

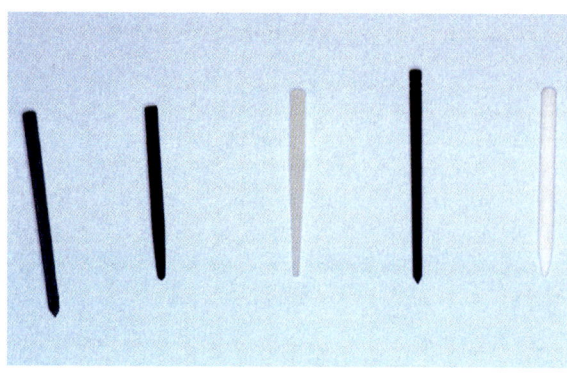

Fig 4-1 (a) Some of the oldest types of fibre posts. From left to right: Aestheti-Plus (quartz fibres, RTD), Endo-Composipost (carbon fibre, RTD), Fiber white (silica fibres, Carbotech), Carbotech (carbon fibres, Carbotech).

Fig 4-1 (b) Glass fibre post featuring retentive grooves for the retention of the composite (Peerless posts, Sybron Endo).

Fig 4-1 (c) Translucent quartz fibre post (DT Light Post, RTD). (d) Radiographic image of glass fibre posts showing an acceptable level of radiopacity.

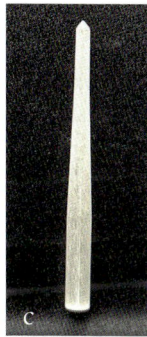

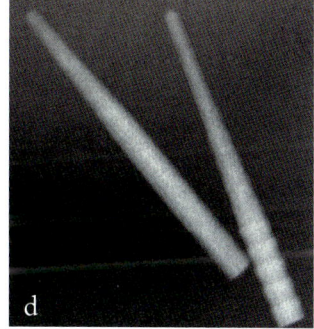

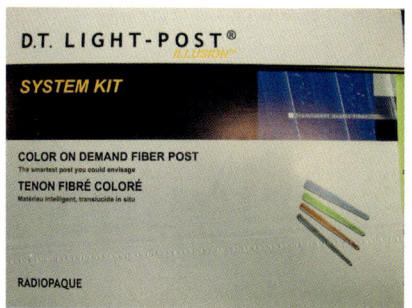

Fig 4-1 (e) The new DT Light Post Illusion (RTD): these posts are colour coded and become translucent at body temperature.

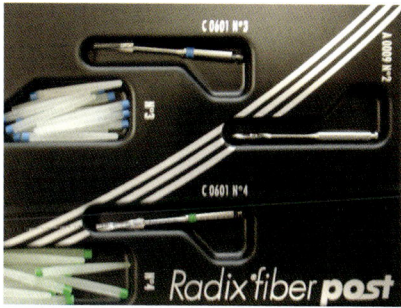

Fig 4-1 (f) The new Radix fibre post (Dentsply Maillefer).

posts, but decementation, which may be associated with marginal leakage and the development of secondary caries.

Adhesion to Composite

The adhesion of the fibre post to composite, as used in a core build-up, is mostly micromechanical, with irregularities on the surface of the post providing retention for the bonding resin (Fig 4-2). Recent work has suggested that silanisation of the post surface may increase the retention of the composite core and adhesion with the luting cement.

Clinical Studies

The clinical evidence supporting the use of fibre posts is abundant and largely superior to that supporting the use of metal posts. At present, no systematic review of randomised clinical studies is available on the restoration of root canal treated teeth using posts.

The vast majority of prospective studies on fibre posts report failure rates in the region of 2 to 5% after 2–5 years of clinical service. Most of the cases reported to have failed did so because of post decementation, chipping of

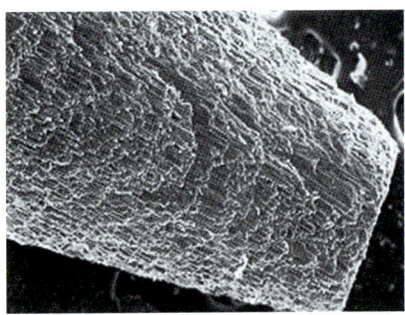

Fig 4-2 (a) SEM image of a fibre post, revealing the roughness that ensures micromechanical bonding to the composite cement.

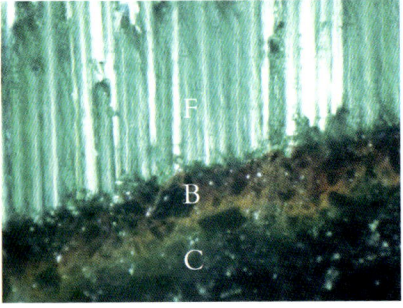

Fig 4-2 (b) Confocal microscopic image showing good adaptation of the bonding system and composite to the post surface: F, fibre post; B, bonding agent; C, composite.

post-supported composite restorations or secondary caries. Only one study reported a high number of post fractures. In none of these studies were teeth lost as a consequence of root fracture. In the only study available on metal posts, a failure rate of 4% was reported. The majority of these failures were found to be caused by root fracture.

Considering the evidence available, it can be concluded that fibre post-composite core restorations are effective in preventing the loss of root canal treated teeth as a consequence of root fracture. Root canal treated teeth restored with fibre post, but not crowned may be at risk of loss of tooth structure through secondary caries.

There is sufficient scientific and clinical evidence to support the use of fibre rather than metal posts in the restoration of root canal treated teeth.

Cementation of Fibre Posts

In the absence of clinical symptoms or a sinus tract, the post-endodontic restoration can be performed at the same visit as the root canal filling.

Single-rooted Teeth
Fibre posts can be used in the restoration of most root canal treated single-rooted teeth. If thin dentinal walls are present, restoration with a fibre post and composite may best preserve the tooth (Fig 4-3). The fibre post limits the risk of root fracture and provides retention for the core. The fibre post will also, together with the composite core, prevent a horizontal fracture of the crown of the tooth.

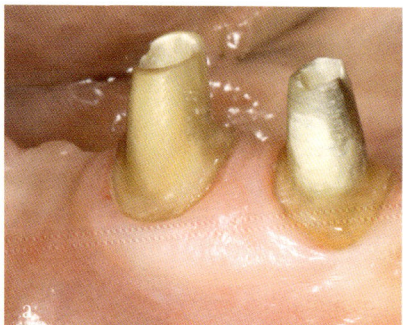 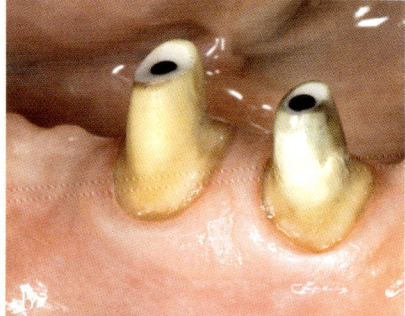

Fig 4-3 (a) and (b) The presence of thin root canal walls is not a contraindication for the use of a fibre post.

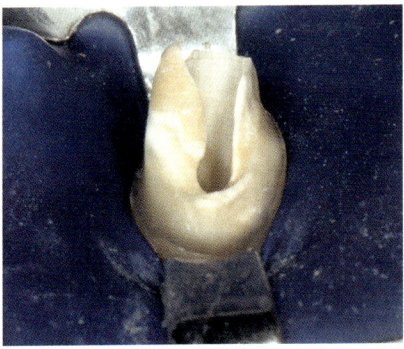

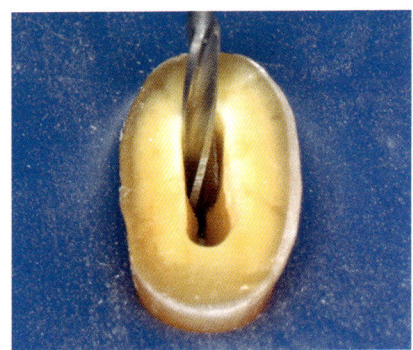

Fig 4-4 The pulp chamber must be thoroughly cleaned before bonding.

Fig 4-5 A Largo drill is used to remove the gutta-percha from the root canal.

Multi-rooted Teeth

- In premolars with two canals, one post is normally sufficient. In maxillary premolars, the palatal canal is normally used for the insertion of the post.
- If a post is needed in molars, one post is normally sufficient. If a deep pulp chamber is available, the use of a post can be avoided. If the residual dentinal walls are thin, two posts may be indicated. Normally, the palatal and distal canals are used in maxillary and mandibular molars respectively. If two posts are needed, the mesio-buccal canal in the maxillary molar and the mesio-lingual in mandibular molars are the canals of choice. In cases of premolarisation or root separation, one post is inserted in each root.

Debridement

If all caries has not been removed prior to the root canal treatment, this should be attended to before restoration. All remnants of gutta-percha, sealer and temporary filling materials must also be removed using sonic tips and magnification (Fig 4-4). Alcohol rinsing to sequester residual eugenol may be indicated.

Re-access and Preparation

Gutta-percha can be removed from the root canal using Gates-Glidden or Largo drills (Fig 4-5). Alternatively, gutta-percha can be removed with heated instruments such as System B (see Chapter 1).

Usually, post-space preparation of a properly filled root canal is limited to a modest enlargement of the coronal third of the root canal, performed using

Gates–Glidden or Largo drills. The use of a bur matching the post is rarely necessary, but if this approach is selected it needs to be done with caution, considering the risk of root perforation. The post chosen is normally the biggest post that reaches the full length of the preparation. The lack of mechanical retention is, in most cases, easily compensated for by the bonding techniques used for the cementation of the post.

Post Length

The post should be at least as long as the clinical crown of the tooth. Shorter posts are at risk of decementation and place the root at risk of fracture. Longer posts may be useful because they increase retention. However, if the root is very long, as in canine teeth, the use of a very long post may increase the risk of preparation perforation and present difficulties if removal becomes necessary. In some cases, the curvature of the root does not allow the use of a long post. In these cases, the use of a fibre post rather than a threaded or other form of active post is indicated if optimal retention is required without increasing the risk of root fracture. An apical gutta–percha seal of 4–5 mm is considered essential for maintaining the integrity of the root filling (Fig 4-6).

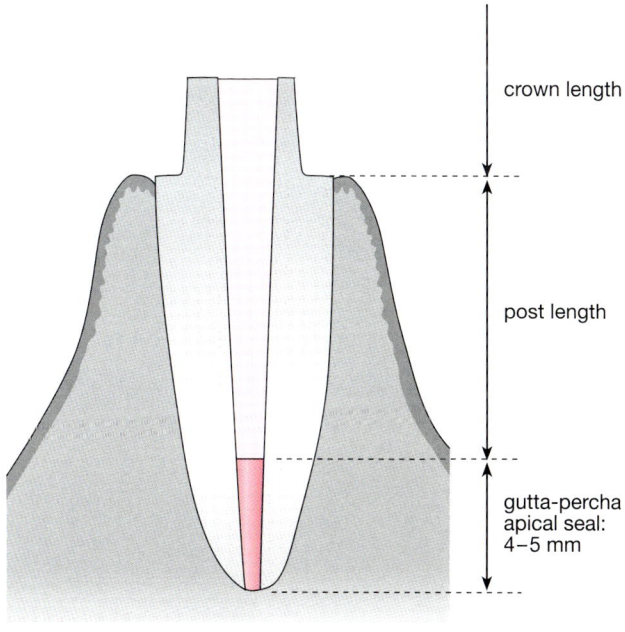

crown length

post length

gutta-percha apical seal: 4–5 mm

Fig 4-6 Schematic illustration of ideal post length.

Isolation

As in all clinical procedures involving an adhesive bonding, rubber dam isolation should be considered routine.

The Use of Matrices

The use of a matrix helps prevent bonding core material to adjacent teeth, as well as enhancing the adaptation of the material to the remaining tooth tissues. The use of a matrix is not essential however, in particular if the core is to be prepared immediately, and there is good access to the preparation.

Bonding

As discussed in Chapter 2, the various forms of existing adhesive systems can be equally effective, assuming use is in strict accordance with manufacturers' directions. The use of a self-etching system reduces the number of steps, as there is no need to wash away the etchant. If the procedure involves washing and drying of the preparation to remove etchant, it is important to use paper points to ensure that the canal is dry prior to the application of the adhesive (Fig 4-7). Long, thin microbrushes should be used to apply the various components of the adhesive system in suitably thin, uniform layers in the post-channel (Fig 4-8). It is important to apply the adhesive to both the post-channel and the post.

Composite Cement

Conventional self- or dual-curing core composites are to be preferred for the cementation of the post and the subsequent core build-up. These materials have mechanical properties close to that of the dentine. Light-curing composites are too thick to be inserted properly into the root canal,

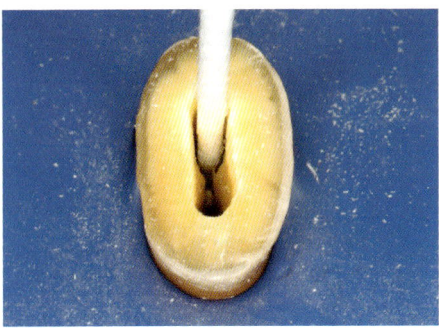

Fig 4-7 Drying the root canal with paper points.

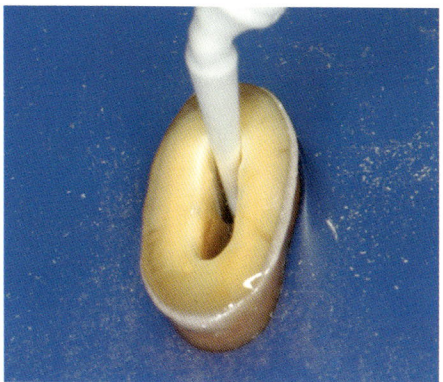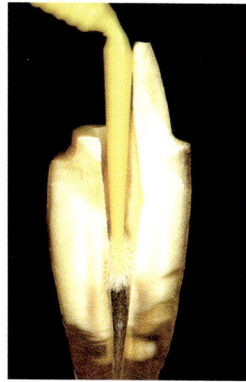

Fig 4-8 Application of bonding resin with microbrushes.

while flowable composites and composite resin cements have a much lower modulus of elasticity and may, therefore, be the weakest part of the restoration. A light-curing system is not used as the fibre post, although translucent, cannot be relied upon to transmit light from the curing unit in sufficient intensity to polymerise the material along the full length of the post-channel.

Insertion of the composite into the root canal
To minimise void formation, the composite cement is injected into the canal with a syringe using specially designed tips (Fig 4-9). Composite is flowed from the base of the post-channel coronally, until the entire post-channel is filled to the brim (Fig 4-10).

Insertion of the Post
The post is immediately inserted into the composite filling the root canal, with no need to place further composite on the post itself.

The Composite Core Build-up
The composite core is added immediately to the newly placed post using the same self-curing composite placed in the post-channel. A light-curing composite may, however, be used to complete the core build-up. It is critical that the post makes no contact with the oral environment and is fully enveloped by composite to avoid the uptake of moisture, which may severely compromise its mechanical behaviour. The crown preparation can, if required, be completed at the same visit.

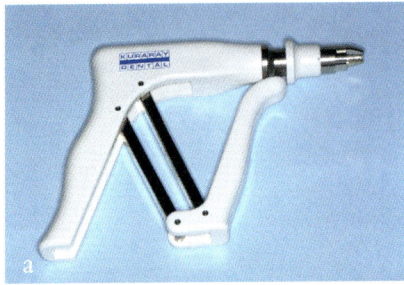
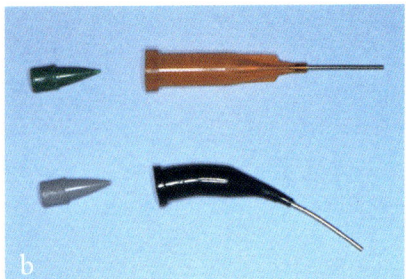
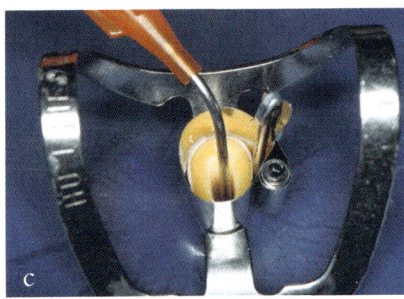

Fig 4-9 Syringe with a specially designed tip for application of self-curing composite to the root canal.

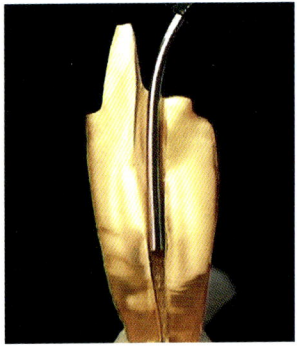

Fig 4-10 Tip designed for the application of composite cement to the full depth of the post-space preparation.

Clinical Sequence of Post Cementation and Crown Build-up (Fig 4-11a-l)

1. Dry the tooth with air and the post-channel with paper points.
2. Apply the self-etching primer to the post-channel and coronal part of the tooth with a microbrush.
3. Gently dry the tooth surface using air and the root canal using paper points.
4. Apply self-curing adhesive to the coronal tissue and post-channel of the tooth, and to the post-surface with a microbrush.

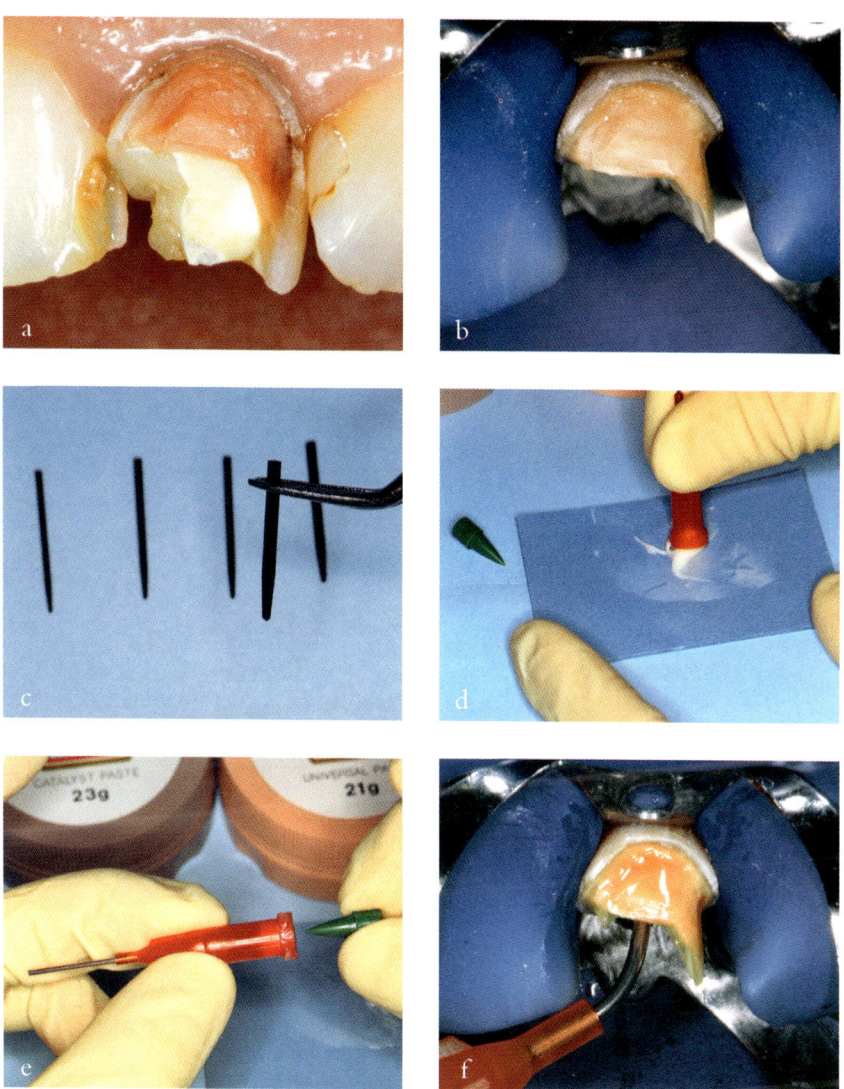

Fig 4-11 Pre-prosthetic restoration: operative sequence (continued over page)

(a) Root-filled upper left central incisor to be restored, in need of restoration with a fibre post and composite core. (b) Tooth isolation with rubber dam. (c) Selection of the fibre post. (d-f) Loading of the composite gun with self-curing composite, and insertion of the composite into the root canal starting from the bottom of the cavity.

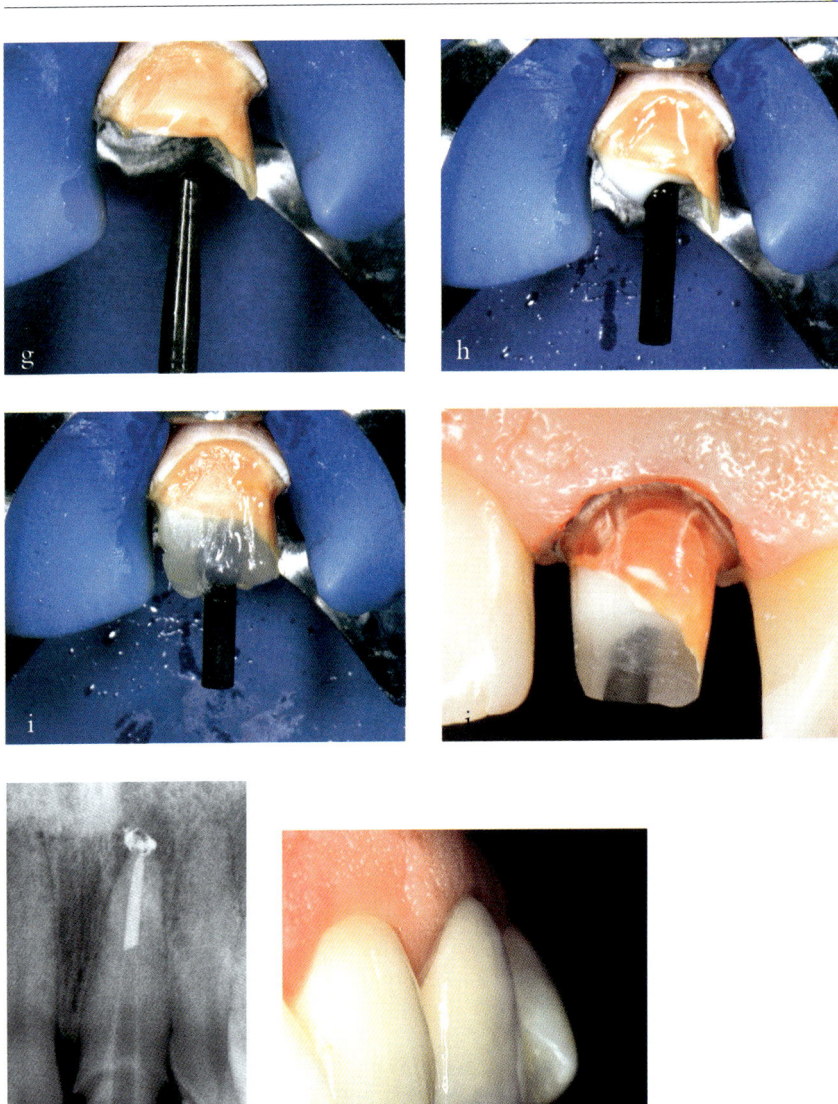

Fig 4-11 Pre-prosthetic restoration: operative sequence (continued)

(g) and (h) Insertion of the post. (i) The core is completed with light-curing composite. (j) Preparation for a crown. (k) Radiograph subsequent to completion of the restoration. The fibre post in this case is radiolucent, but the radiopaque cement clearly reveals the outline of the post. (l) All-ceramic crown following cementation (In-Ceram, Vita, Germany).

5. Remove excess bonding resin from the tooth surface and post-channel with an air syringe and paper points.
6. Mix the self-curing composite.
7. Insert the composite into the syringe tip.
8. Apply the tip to the syringe.
9. Insert the tip into the deepest part of the post preparation and backfill with composite resin.
10. Insert the post.
11. Start the core build-up using the remaining self-curing composite. If needed, a light-curing composite can be used to complete the crown build-up, following 4–5 minutes to allow complete setting of the self-curing composite.

Further Reading

Duret B, Reynaud M, Duret F. Un nouveau concept de reconstitution corono-radiculaire: le Composipost. Le Chirurgian Dentiste de France 1990;540:31–141.

Glazer B. Restoration of endodontically treated teeth with carbon fibre posts – a prospective study. J Canadian Dent Assoc 2000;66:613-618.

Grandini S, Goracci C, Tay FR, Grandini R, Ferrari M. Clinical evaluation of the use of fiber posts and direct resin restorations for endodontically treated teeth. Int J Prosthodontics 2005;18:399–404.

Malferrari S, Monaco C, Scotti R. Clinical evaluation of teeth restored with quartz fiber-reinforced epoxy resin posts. Int J Prosthodontics 2003;16:39–44.

Mannocci F, Bertelli E, Sherriff M, Watson TF, Pitt Ford TR. Three-year clinical comparison of survival of endodontically treated teeth restored with either full cast coverage or with direct composite restoration. J Prosthetic Dent 2002;88:297–301.

Mannocci F, Qualtrough AJ, Worthington HV, Watson TF, Pitt Ford TR. Randomized clinical comparison of endodontically treated teeth restored with amalgam or with fiber posts and resin composite: five-year results. Oper Dent 2005;30:9–15.

Monticelli F, Grandini S, Goracci C, Ferrari M. Clinical behaviour of translucent-fiber posts: a 2-year prospective study. Int J Prosthodontics 2003;16:593–596.

Naumann M, Blankenstein F, Dietrich T. Survival of glass fibre reinforced composite post restorations after 2 years – an observational clinical study. J Dent 2005;33:305–312.

Chapter 5

Problem Solving in the Restoration of Teeth with Fibre Posts

Aim

To describe how to make a customised fibre post that will adapt to a root canal of irregular shape and how to use interpenetrating polymer network (IPN) glass fibre posts.

Outcome

At the end of this chapter, the reader should understand how to make a customised fibre post-composite core restoration and to use IPN glass fibre posts.

Introduction

The vast majority of root canals have an irregular, ovoid shape in their coronal and middle thirds, elements of which may remain following preparation. The consequent lack of adaptation of the post to the root canal walls may compromise the ability of the luting agent to completely fill the post–tooth interface completely. This might be associated with decementation of the post.

If a decision is made to cement a post into a root canal, the risk of void spaces within the root canal should be minimised.

The problem of the discrepancy between the irregular cross section of the root canal and the circular cross section of the post may be difficult to solve, in particular in teeth that have undergone an endodontic retreatment including the removal of a customised cast post (Fig 5-1a,b). The preparation for the cast post and core, followed by the removal of the post often results in a wide root canal space.

Similar problems tend to be created in preparation of short roots or by the presence of severe curvatures within roots. If the length of root available for bonding is limited, the adaptation of the composite to the root canal walls

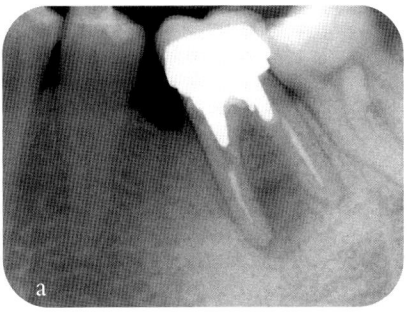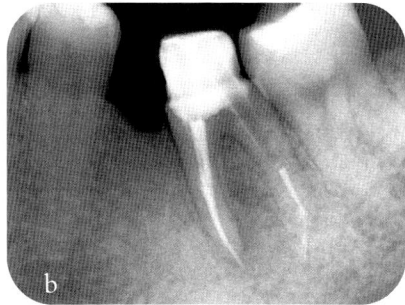

Fig 5-1 (a) and (b) The lower left second molar shows a periapical radiolucency associated with an existing root canal treatment and a cast post. After removing the cast post and root canal retreatment, the tooth was re-restored with a fibre post and composite core.

must be optimised. Critical are the size and number of voids present in the layer of bonding resin and cement, which may weaken the bond between the various components of the tooth–restoration complex (dentine, bonding agent, composite, post).

Customising Fibre Posts

The adhesion of composite resin to a fibre post can be used to create a fibre post-composite core perfectly adapted to the shape of irregular root canals.

Steps required for the construction of such a fibre post customised with composite are as follows:
1. Complete the root canal treatment or retreatment (Fig 5-2a,b).
2. Remove the root canal filling material to the desired level. An endodontic probe and a heating ultrasonic tip used under magnification are useful adjuncts in this process.
3. The widest fibre post that extends the full depth of the post-space preparation is selected.
4. A bonding agent is applied to the post surface and gently spread with compressed air to ensure complete wetting (Fig 5-2c).
5. The bonding agent is cured for 60 s.
6. A dual curing composite is then applied to the post surface.
7. The composite-covered post is inserted into the post-channel.

Fig 5-2 (a) and (b) The upper right canine is associated with a periapical radiolucency despite an existing root canal treatment. After post removal, the root canal treatment is completed.

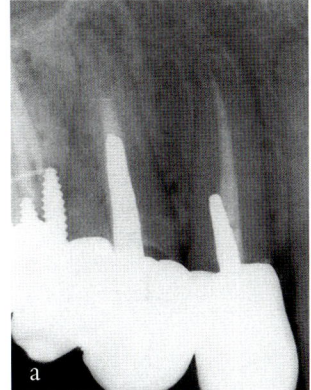 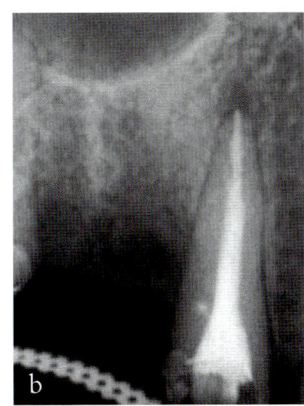

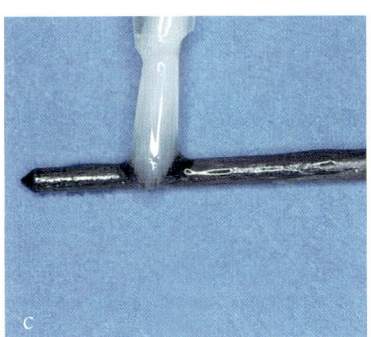 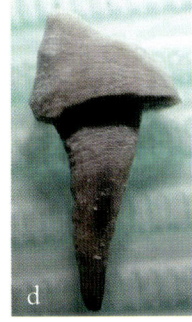 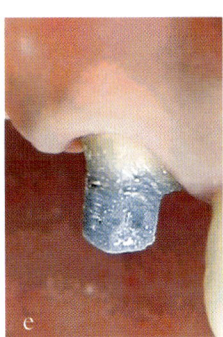

Fig 5-2 (c)–(e) Construction and cementation of a customised fibre post.

8. Once the composite has passed initial set, it is carefully withdrawn, and the surface inspected for the presence of voids (Fig 5-2d).
9. Further composite is added in areas of deficiency, before re-inserting the post to capture an "impression" of the canal space.
10. The composite-covered post is removed once again and then cemented into the root canal using a dual-cure cement.
11. The core is then built and shaped (Fig 5-2e).

Sections of roots which contain posts cemented by the conventional (Fig 5-3a) and customised technique (Fig 5-3b) reveal important differences. It is evident that the latter technique allows a void-free cementation, whereas a large void is present within the cement layer in the case managed using a conventional technique.

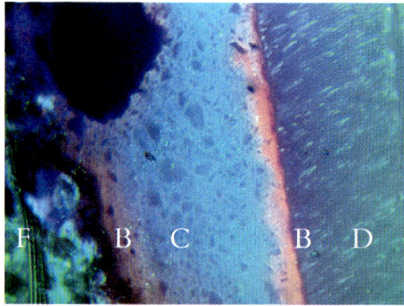

Fig 5-3 (a) Confocal microscopic image of a fibre post cemented into a root canal by a conventional technique. A large void is evident within the cement layer. (F, fibre post; B, bonding resin; C, composite cement; D, dentine).

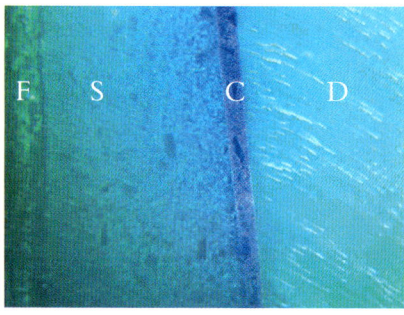

Fig 5-3 (b) Confocal microscopic image of a customised fibre post cemented into the root canal: no voids are noted (F, fibre post; S, composite core; C, composite cement; D, dentine).

IPN Fibre Posts

IPN posts are made of glass fibres immersed in an unpolymerised resin matrix. The monomers of the bonding resin diffuse into the linear phases of the IPN polymer matrix and after polymerisation interlock the fibres.

By using IPN posts, it is possible to adapt the post to the shape of the root canals and to obtain excellent bonding between the post, the bonding resin and the composite cement. This helps prevent decementation of the post and debonding of the composite core from the post.

Clinical Case

A seven-year-old boy was referred after an accident in which his maxillary central incisor was fractured and the pulp exposed (Fig 5-4a,b). The pulp was irreversibly inflamed. The tooth fragment was preserved in sterile saline solution for six months, then his parents were instructed to change the saline on a daily basis. After apicogenesis of the tooth was achieved by the application of calcium hydroxide, an IPN fibre post (Fig 5-4c), in combination with a self-curing bonding system and composite, was used to rebond the fragment to the tooth (Fig 5-4d-g).

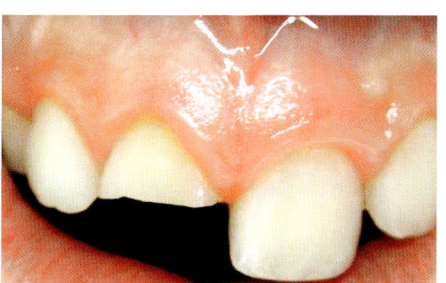

Fig 5-4 (a) Fractured upper right central incisor in a seven-year-old child.

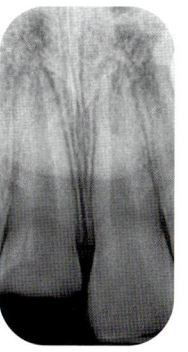

Fig 5-4 (b) Radiographic image of the tooth showing an open root apex.

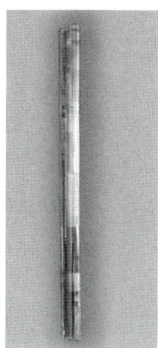

Fig 5-4 (c) IPN post used for the restoration of the tooth.

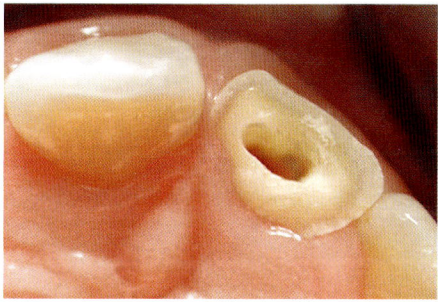

Fig 5-4 (d) Palatal view of the tooth after the root canal treatment.

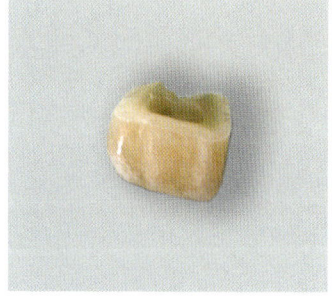

Fig 5-4 (e) The tooth fragment is ready for rebonding.

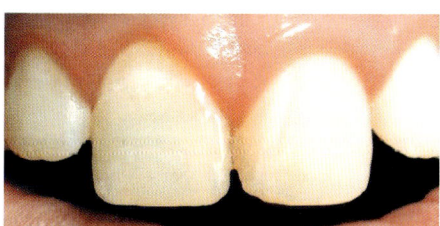

Fig 5-4 (f) After apicogenesis, the tooth fragment has been reattached using an IPN post and bonding agent with self-curing composite.

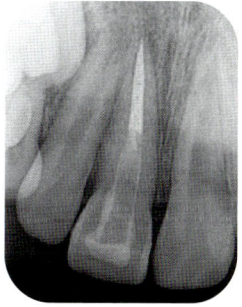

Fig 5-4 (g) Post-restorative radiograph.

Further Reading

Cantatore G. L'Anatomia canalare e le tecniche di ricostruzione post-endodontica. Atti del II° Simposio Internazionale "Odontoiatria Adesiva Oggi". S. Margherita Ligure 20–21 Marzo 1998. 1998 Hippocrates Ed. Medico Scientifiche S.r.l.-Milano.

Kallio T, Lastumäki T, Vallittu PK. Bonding of restorative composite resin to some polymeric composite substrates. Dent Mater J 2001;17:80–86.

Lastumäki TM, Kallio TT, Vallittu PK. The bond strength of light-curing composite resin to finally polymerized and aged glass fiber–reinforced composite substrate. Biomaterials 2002;23:4533-4539.

Lastumäki TM, Lassila LVJ, Vallittu PK. The semi-interpenetrating polymer network matrix of fiber–reinforced composite and its effect on the surface adhesive properties. J Material Sci Mater Med 2003;14:803-809.

Chapter 6

Understanding the Failure of Adhesive Restorations in Root Canal Treated Teeth

Aim

To describe the causes of failure of adhesive restorations in root canal treated teeth.

Outcome

At the end of this chapter, the reader should be able to understand the reasons why adhesive restorations fail in root canal treated teeth, and know how to predictably re-restore them.

Failures

Post-core Decementation
- Decementation is the primary cause of restoration failure in teeth restored with fibre posts, composite cores and metal-ceramic crowns. This is caused mainly by the degradation of the dentine–composite bond under the influence of function and components of the oral environment. When fibre posts make any contact with oral fluids, their flexural strength is greatly reduced, and this combined with cyclic loading plays an important part in causing the post-core decementation. Post-core decementation is often associated with secondary caries (Fig 6-1).

How to minimise the risks of post-core decementation
- Carefully evaluate the amount of tooth structure available, considering also the amount of tooth structure that will be lost as a result of any subsequent crown preparation. A lack of coronal tooth structure available for bonding is one of the main causes of decementation.
- Carefully consider if a crown is indicated or not. Research has shown that in anterior teeth, crowning may not increase the likelihood of tooth survival (see Chapter 3). Research has also shown that decementation of the post is highly unlikely to happen if the tooth has not been prepared for a crown. In short, in anterior teeth, post placement and crowning is indicated only if a complete loss of crown tooth structure

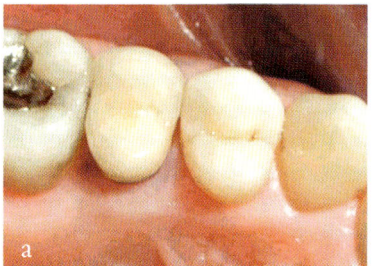
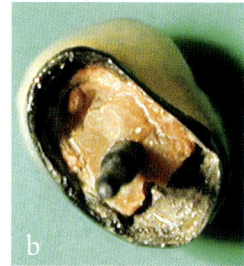
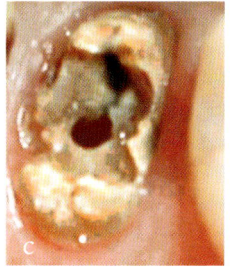
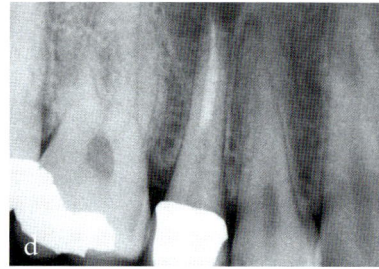

Fig 6-1 Post-core decementation associated with secondary caries (b-c) and a periapical radiolucency (d).

is present, or if the aesthetic requirements of the patient cannot be met otherwise.

- The presence of bruxism or other parafunctions may cause failure of post-core restorations. Night guards may be of some help, but the patient needs to be aware that all restorations are at risk of failure when subjected to parafunctions.
- Preserve as much coronal tooth tissue as possible.
- Ensure that a proper ferrule has been developed.
- Ensure that the maximum possible length of the post-space preparation has been created, without risking root perforation or compromising the seal of the root canal filling.
- Choose the appropriate post size.
- Isolate the tooth with a rubber dam for moisture control and optimal bonding to dentine.
- Remove all the remnants of gutta-percha and sealer from the root canal space using an endodontic explorer, under magnification, to optimise the dentinal surface available for the bonding.
- Rinse the canal with absolute alcohol to sequester any residual eugenol if eugenol-containing materials have been employed.
- Use a customised post-core if a significant discrepancy exists between the morphology of the root canals and that of the post (see Chapter 5).

Procedure for the management of post-core decementations

Carefully evaluate if the tooth is re-restorable – see Chapter 8 for the decision-making process on the restorability of root canal treated teeth. If the tooth is re-restorable, the best option would normally be to make a new fibre post and composite core before constructing a new crown. If it is agreed with the patient not to start again, it may be possible to simply recement the post-core and crown as follows:

- Working with magnification and ultrasound, carefully remove all remnants of composite and bonding agent from the root canal.
- Attempt to reposition the post-crown, checking its marginal adaptation and occlusal relationships.
- If the post-crown appears satisfactory, isolate the tooth.
- Etch the root canal for 40 s.
- Introduce a dual curing, self-etching priming composite cement into the root canal and onto the post (Fig 6-2).
- Introduce the post-crown into the root canal.

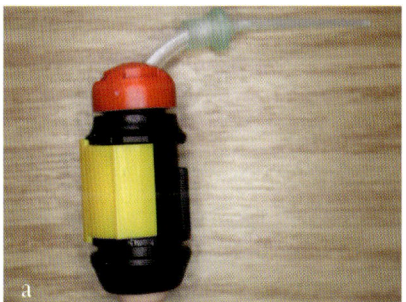
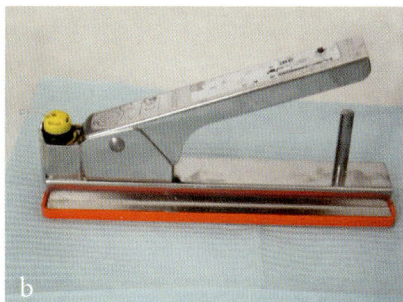
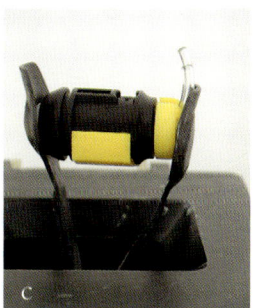
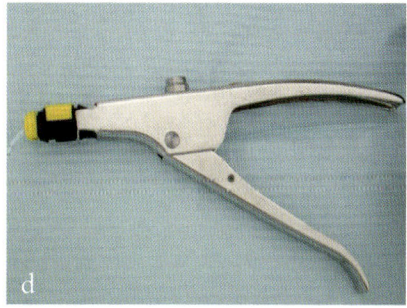

Fig 6-2 (a) A resin cement capsule featuring a special tip for the insertion of the composite cement into the root canal. The capsule needs to be activated (b), mixed for 15–20 s (c) and inserted into the gun (d). The cement is then applied into the root canal.

- Carefully remove any excess composite cement before it is fully cured.
- Carefully adjust the occlusion.

Detachment of the Composite Core-crown

Detachment of the composite core-crown from the post is a very rare complication. This may happen when no coronal tooth structure is left and a post has been used to support a long clinical crown. Contamination of the post surface during the bonding procedure and lack of attention to detail may also cause this type of failure. The risk of this type of failure may, in addition to meticulous attention to detail, be reduced by the presence of a ferrule.

The ideal management of a composite core-crown detachment is the construction of a new composite core, followed by a replacement crown. If, after discussion with the patient, it is agreed that the existing crown is to be reused, a new core may be created as follows (Fig 6-3):
- Carefully remove the composite from the interior of the crown using an ultrasonic tip and/or a carbide bur mounted on a high-speed handpiece. Ensure that any water spray is free from oily contamination.

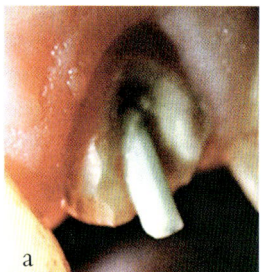
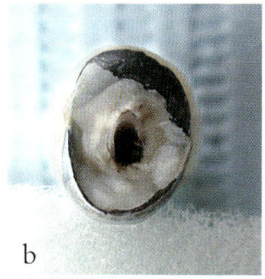
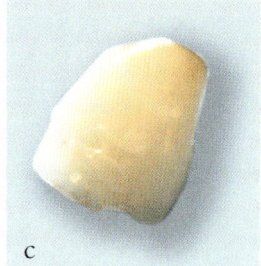

a

b

c

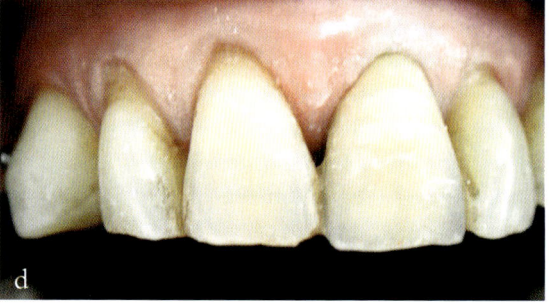

d

Fig 6-3 The composite core and crown detached from a post cemented into an upper left central incisor. The composite core was reconstructed and the crown recemented.

- Isolate the tooth with a rubber dam.
- Apply a self-curing bonding agent to the post.
- Apply a separating medium, such as petroleum jelly, to the interior of the crown.
- Pack self-curing composite resin around the post in the form of a new core. Care is needed to ensure that only limited excess is applied.
- Reposition the crown on the freshly placed composite core.
- Remove the crown as soon as the composite has polymerised.
- Remove composite excesses from the core and crown.
- Reposition the crown to check seating and occlusion.
- Recement the crown.

Fibre Post Fracture

- The literature on fibre post restorations indicates that post fracture is uncommon.
- The main cause is usually the use of a post which is too narrow for its intended purpose in the restoration of a severely compromised tooth which is subjected to heavy occlusal loading (Fig 6-4).

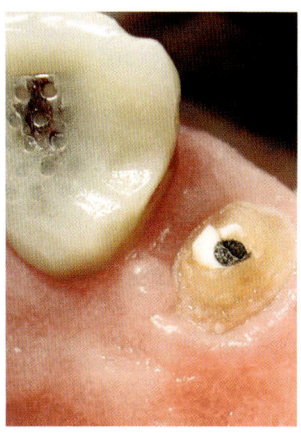

Fig 6-4 A fractured carbon fibre post.

The risk of post fracture may be minimised by:

- Carefully evaluating the amount of residual tooth structure left and considering other alternatives for the restoration of, in particular, a severely damaged tooth.
- Repeating the root canal treatment if the root canal preparation appears to be insufficient for the placement of a post of appropriate size.
- Using tried and tested fibre post systems.

Management of a fractured fibre post

- Carefully evaluate the amount of residual tooth structure left and consider whether the tooth is restorable.
- If the tooth is considered restorable, remove the fractured fragment of the post from the root canal (see Chapter 7).
- Using ultrasonic or sonic vibratory devices and magnification, remove all of remaining composite material from the root canal.
- Carefully enlarge the post–space.
- Cement a new post, construct a new core and recrown the tooth.

Root Fracture

Clinical studies indicate that root fractures are rare in teeth restored with fibre posts, composite cores and crowns. Root fractures may be associated with post decementation in severely compromised teeth, for which the prognosis would be poor whichever restorative method is employed. The inherent flexibility of fibre posts promotes failure by debond rather than root fracture. This should be viewed as an advantage of fibre post approaches to the treatment of root canal treated teeth.

The risk of root fracture may be minimised in a number of ways including:
- Only teeth with at least 2 mm of coronal dentine should be considered realistic candidates for successful post-core and crown restoration.
- Ideally, roots should be checked under magnification before restoration to exclude evidence of root fracture.
- Endodontic procedures should be conducted in such a way as to minimise the transfer of damaging loads to teeth and to minimise dentine removal as far as possible, consistent with high-quality treatment.
- The occlusion of all restorations should be checked with care, in particular in patients with parafunctions.
- Posts should be as long as possible, without compromising the root filling or tooth, to maximally distribute occlusally generated stresses.
- Post-channels should not be unnecessarily enlarged at the cost of structurally important dentine.

Treatment of root fractures
- If the root fracture occurs above the level of the periodontal attachment, the tooth can be re-restored, usually using a composite restoration that replaces the missing tooth structure.
- If the root fracture occurs below the level of the periodontal attachment, it may be possible to recover the tooth by surgical crown lengthening or orthodontic forced eruption, but if the fracture is too deeply located, extraction is the only option.

Failure of Intracoronal Restorations

Several short- and long-term clinical studies have highlighted that teeth restored with fibre posts and composite have different failure modes to teeth restored with fibre posts, composite cores and crowns. The most common failure modes are:
- secondary caries   • chipping of the composite
- fracture of the root (extremely rare).

The Risk of Secondary Caries May Be Reduced By:

- Ensuring that the patient is aware of the maintenance needs of their complex restorations and by providing an appropriate package of maintenance care, including detailed oral hygiene and dietary instruction.
- Considering the possibility of crowning the tooth if the amount of remaining tooth is limited; clinical studies of crowned teeth report a very low incidence of secondary caries.
- Carefully isolating the tooth by means of the rubber dam prior to restoration.
- Keeping the margins of the restoration in areas where they are accessible for oral hygiene maintenance – crown lengthening procedures may be necessary in some circumstances.
- Ensuring properly contoured restorations to promote optimal plaque control.

In the event of secondary caries requiring operative intervention, caries removal and re-restoration of the tooth tends to be followed by crown coverage. Crown lengthening procedures may be needed if the caries are subgingival.

Chipping

Chipping of a composite is normally a minor problem that is simply solved by repair or, if extensive, replacement of the composite. Normally, the presence of the fibre post ensures sufficient support to the new composite restoration. However, the placement of a crown is often indicated if the composite is large and suffers repeated chipping (Fig 6-5).

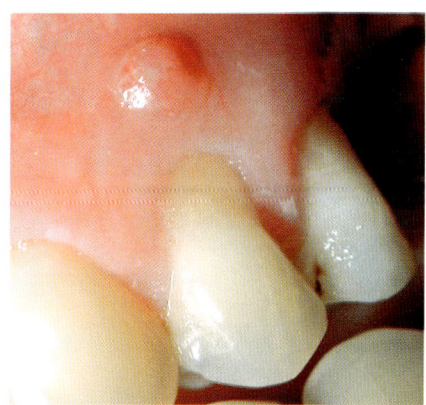

Fig 6-5 (a) A sinus tract is present on the buccal aspect of an upper right first premolar (continued over page).

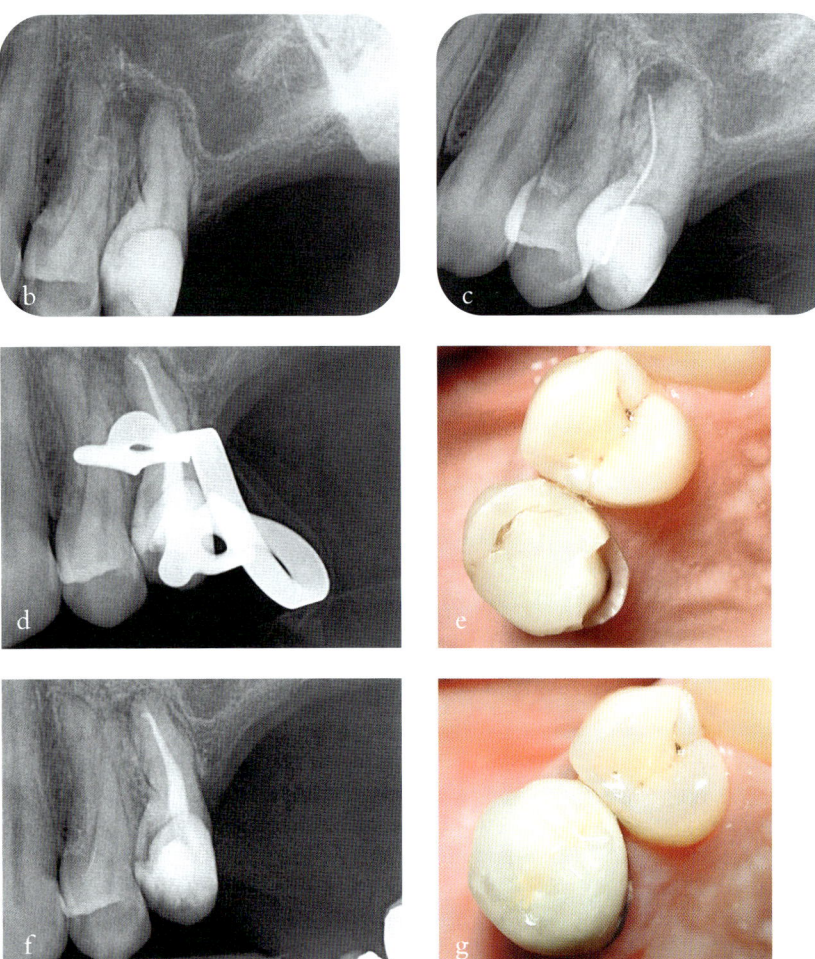

Fig 6-5 (b-g) Radiographic examination revealed that the sinus tract originated for the upper right second premolar (b) and (c). The root canal treatment was completed (d) and the tooth restored with composite resin. At a two-year recall, chipping of the composite restoration was observed (e). The periapical radiolucency had healed (f). The tooth was restored with a metal-ceramic crown.

Fracture of the Root

Fracture of the root is relatively rare. The causes and the treatment procedure are similar to those described for post-core-crown adhesive restorations of root canal treated teeth. The lack of cusp coverage may be associated with root fractures (Fig 6-6).

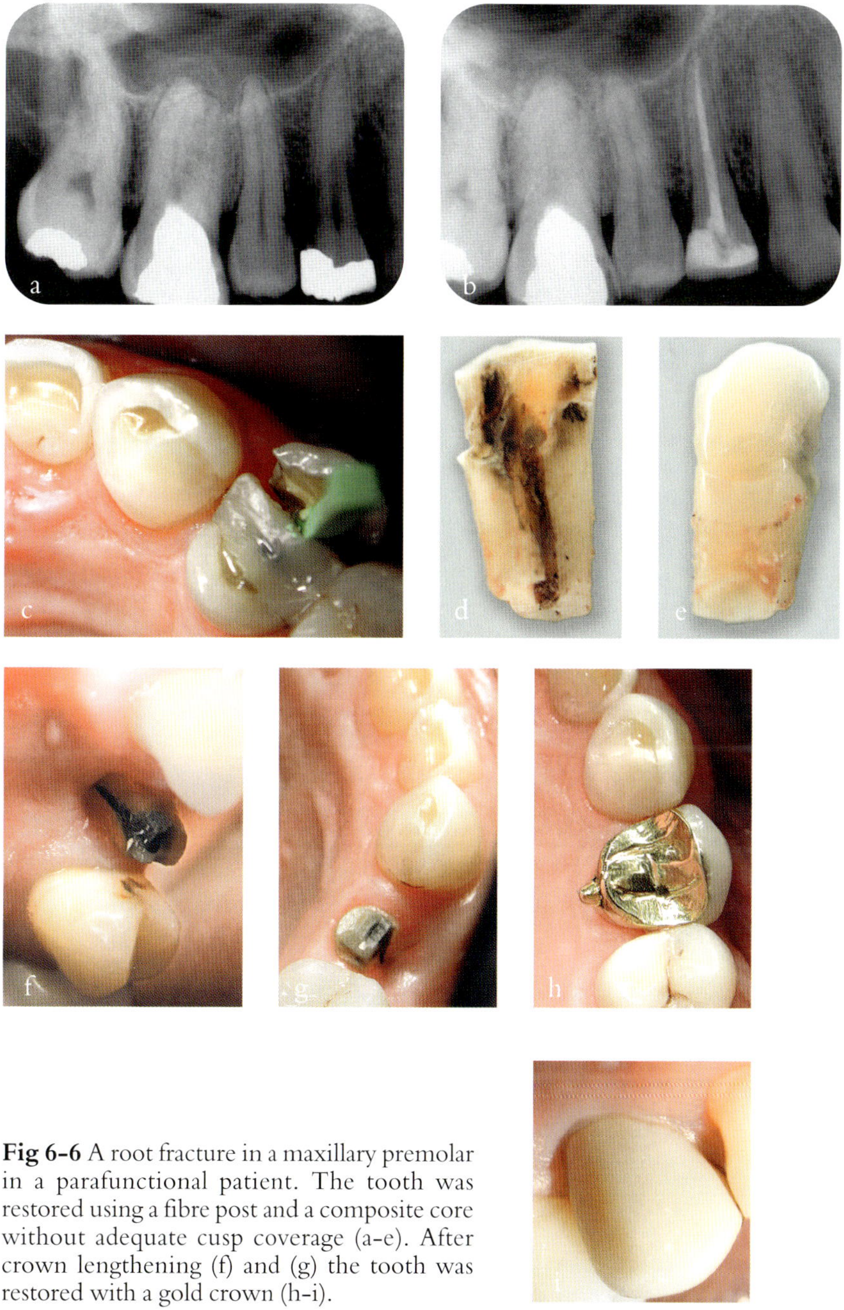

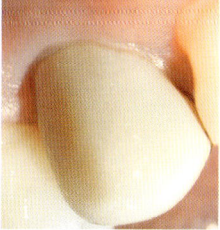

Fig 6-6 A root fracture in a maxillary premolar in a parafunctional patient. The tooth was restored using a fibre post and a composite core without adequate cusp coverage (a-e). After crown lengthening (f) and (g) the tooth was restored with a gold crown (h-i).

Further Reading

Glazer B. Restoration of endodontically treated teeth with carbon fibre posts – a prospective study. J Canadian Dent Assoc 2000;66:613–618.

Grandini S, Goracci C, Tay FR, Grandini R, Ferrari M. Clinical evaluation of the use of fiber posts and direct resin restorations for endodontically treated teeth. Int J Prosthodontics 2005;18:399–404.

King PA, Setchell DJ, Rees JS. Clinical evaluation of a carbon fibre reinforced carbon endodontic post. J Oral Rehabil 2003;30:785–789.

Malferrari S, Monaco C, Scotti R. Clinical evaluation of teeth restored with quartz fiber-reinforced epoxy resin posts. Int J Prosthodontics 2003;16: 39–44.

Mannocci F, Bertelli E, Sherriff M, Watson TF, Ford TR. Three-year clinical comparison of survival of endodontically treated teeth restored with either full cast coverage or with direct composite restoration. J Prosthetic Dent 2002;88:297–301.

Mannocci F, Bertelli E, Watson TF, Pitt Ford TR. *Ex vivo* study of resin-dentin interfaces of endodontically-treated restored teeth. Am J Dent 2003;16:28–32.

Mannocci F, Qualtrough AJ, Worthington HV, Watson TF, Pitt Ford TR. Randomized clinical comparison of endodontically treated teeth restored with amalgam or with fiber posts and resin composite: five-year results. Oper Dent 2005;30:9–15.

Monticelli F, Grandini S, Goracci C, Ferrari M. Clinical behaviour of translucent-fibre posts: a 2-year prospective study. Int J Prosthodontics 2003;16:593–596.

Naumann M, Blankenstein F, Dietrich T. Survival of glass fibre reinforced composite post restorations after 2 years – an observational clinical study. J Dent 2005;33:305–312.

Chapter 7

Endodontic Retreatment of Teeth Restored with Adhesive Techniques and Fibre Posts

Aim

To describe the procedure for the removal of a cemented fibre post from the root canal.

Outcome

At the end of this chapter, the reader should be able to identify the risks and be knowledgeable on methods for the removal of fibre posts from root canals.

Introduction

The term "post-treatment disease" includes all persistent, recurrent and emerged apical periodontitis associated with endodontically treated teeth (Fig 7-1a-c). This condition, caused by microbial infection of the root canal system, is frequently associated with a periapical radiolucency. It affects between 5-35% of root canal treated teeth.

Coronal leakage associated with secondary caries, debond and loss of coronal restorations is often implicated in post-treatment endodontic disease. After removal of defective restorations and secondary caries, an endodontic retreatment is often attempted in order to eliminate infection from the root canal space.

Post removal is often considered a major challenge to endodontic retreatment, in particular if the post is bonded with adhesive cement. Added to this, few practitioners have experience of fibre post removal, and the challenge is often considered to be daunting.

Diagnosis

Radiographic identification of contemporary fibre posts is straightforward, but earlier, radiolucent posts may be difficult to identify. Under such a

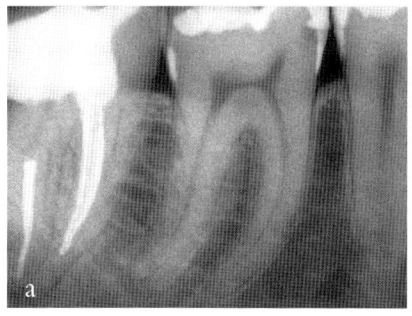
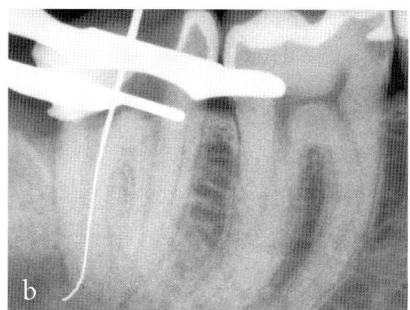
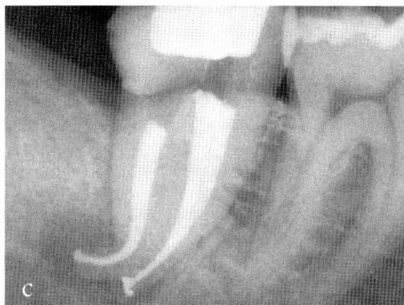

Fig 7-1 (a) A lower right second molar affected by post-endodontic disease: note the fibre post inserted in the distal root. (b) After removal of the fibre post, the canal is negotiated and the working length determined. (c) Awaiting final coronal restoration.

circumstance, an apparently empty canal may be surrounded by a thin, radiopaque line of resin cement.

A decision must often be made whether to remove the crown or work through it. Working through a crown may present special challenges, since instruments will need to be inserted along the long axis of the post to be removed, and this may be impossible through a conservative coronal access. Although the canal which contains the post may be readily identified, other canals which may also need retreatment may be difficult to identify within a mass of tooth-coloured composite, in a deep cavity.

The wise option is usually to remove the crown as part of the package of care.

Armamentarium
As with many procedures in dentistry, the correct tools are helpful. These may include:
- instrumentation for crown and bridge removal

- magnification
- rotary instruments
- ultrasonic equipment and tips.

Magnification aids include simple loupes, with or without supplementary lighting, and operating microscopes (Figs 7-2 to 7-5). An operating microscope greatly facilitates retreatments.

Microscopes have not yet become established in mainstream general practice, owing largely to the capital cost, but also to the training and familiarisation

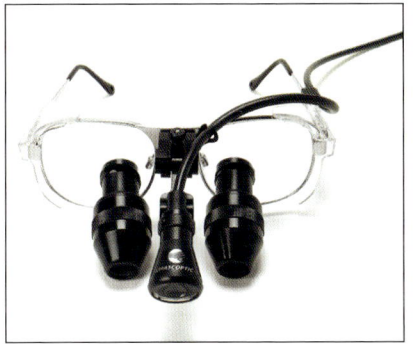

Fig 7-2 Loupes with an LED lamp.

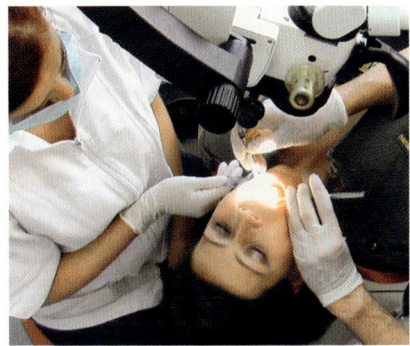

Fig 7-3 A typical session of endodontic microintervention.

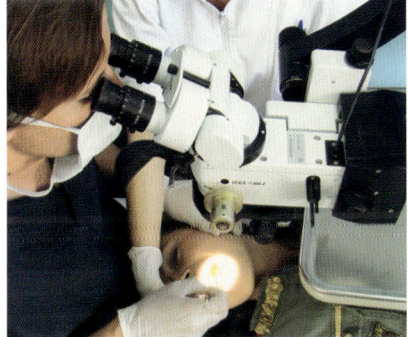

Fig 7-4 Optimal positioning of operator, assistant and patient while working on a lower tooth under magnification.

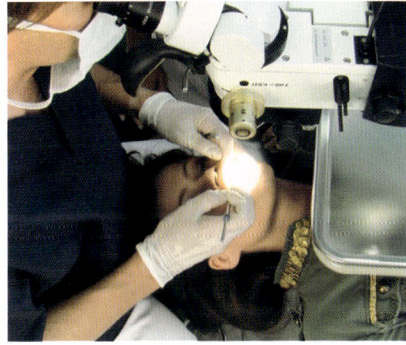

Fig 7-5 Positioning for a maxillary tooth.

required by both the dentist and the chair-side personnel. Loupes are, however, widely employed in practice.

Working with magnification
Operator position, patient position and role of the dental nurse may be altered in practices which adopt magnification.

Working with a microscope, the operator position of choice is usually behind the patient's head, in the "12 o'clock" position. The patient may be supported in neck extension, in particular when working on lower teeth. The dental nurse needs her own binocular and should be trained in "four-handed work under magnification".

Principles of Post Removal
Unlike metallic posts, fibre posts are not readily removed by simple lute-disruption: by means of ultrasonic and pulling techniques. Fibre posts must be cut out with burs and the use of ultrasonics which are advanced along the "grain" of the post, separating the fibres from their resinous matrix.

Rotary instruments
A variety of long-shanked burs are available for the removal of fibre posts. Long-shanked burs keep the head of the handpiece out of the dentist's line of vision and burs with narrow shanks, such as goose-neck and long-necked pin burs, allow close watch to be kept on the bur head (Figs 7-6 and 7-7).

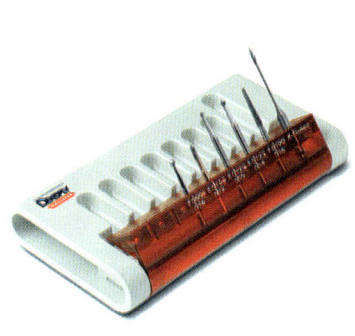

Fig 7-6 A set of long-shank burs.

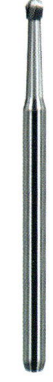

Fig 7-7 A long-shank tungsten-carbide round bur, ideal to remove decayed tissue under magnification.

Gates-Glidden and modified Gates-Glidden "belly" burs are also suitable for such applications.

These instruments can be used with or without water cooling, provided that care is taken not to allow aggressive bur application and overheating deep in the canal. Intermittent washing and drying of the dentinal surface also helps distinguish between composite resin and dentine.

Ultrasonic devices
A variety of steel and diamond-coated ultrasonic tips are available to cut dental materials and tooth tissue. Most are driven by powerful piezoelectric ultrasonic units (Figs 7-8 to 7-10). Their cutting is not as efficient as a high-speed diamond bur, but their vibratory motion allows composite resin to be carefully detached from dentine, ideally under the control of magnification. Any risk of tooth perforation is also reduced, though great care should be exercised.

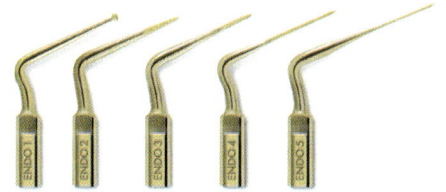

Fig 7-8 A series of ultrasonic endodontic tips.

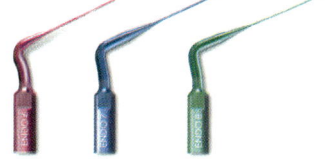

Fig 7-9 A series of ultrasonic diamond-coated endodontic tips.

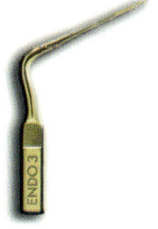

Fig 7-10 A single ultrasonic endodontic tip: note the diamond coating distribution to enhance cutting ability.

Procedure

In the event that a coronal restoration has fractured or become detached from the post, identification of the post should not be challenging.

If the coronal restoration remains intact, the crown should first be removed by conventional means, taking steps to ensure that materials and some form of matrix are available to construct a satisfactory provisional restoration.

- Following crown removal (Fig 7-11), the composite core is first cleaned and inspected to identify the head of the post. (Fig 7-12a,b).

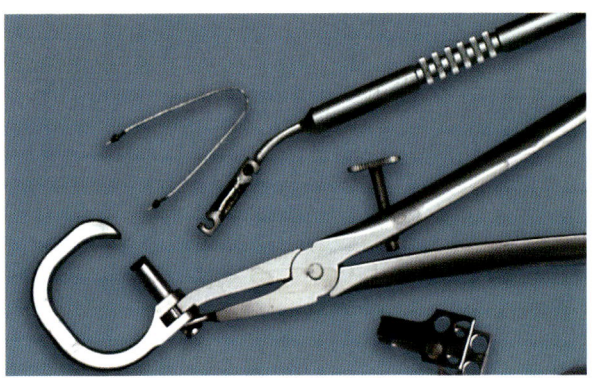

Fig 7-11 A system to remove crown and bridges.

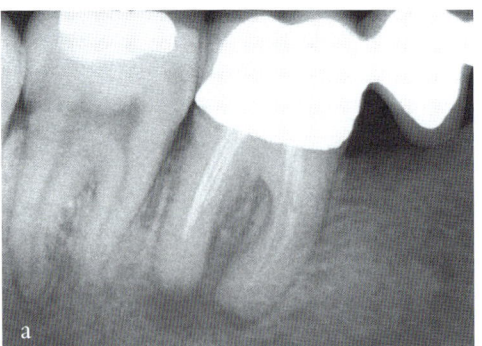
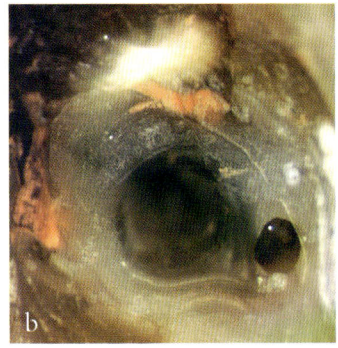

Fig 7-12 (a) Post-endodontic disease affecting a lower right first molar including a fibre post. (b) After disassembling the prosthetic crown, a large mass of composite is found to surround the post in the distal root (continued on pages 95 and 96).

- If the head of the post is not apparent, it is probably contained within the composite core, and judicious shortening of the composite core should be undertaken to identify the post. First generation "carbon fibre" posts are black and very readily identified. Many quartz and glass-fibre posts are translucent or grey and may again be readily identified. Occasionally, posts may be difficult to differentiate from the surrounding composite without magnification.

  Once identified, the removal of a fibre post involves drilling up its centre with a bur, which will soften the post matrix and disrupt its fibres. Diamond-coated burs are often more effective than Gates-Glidden burs in drilling through the post structure.

Great care should be exercised to ensure correct long-axis orientation. Periodic checking with good light and magnification is advised. Progress is usually rapid as the post disrupts ahead of the bur. Particular care should be exercised in the depths of the post-channel:
- to remove the deepest part of the post in the most slender part of the root without perforation or other damage
- to disrupt the pool of composite cement which may block further progress of endodontic retreatment after post removal.

Fine ultrasonically energised tips are often essential for both of these tasks, and again, ideally under the control of magnification and good lighting (Fig 7-12c-j).

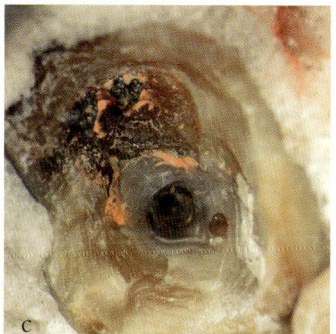 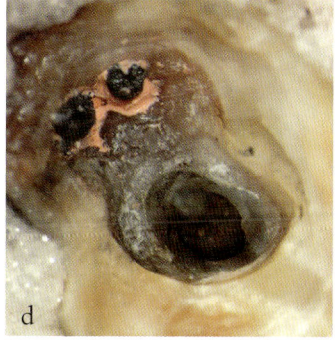

Fig 7-12 (c) Careful work with ultrasonic tips to remove resin from the mesial part of the tooth. (d) Isolation of the post (continued over page).

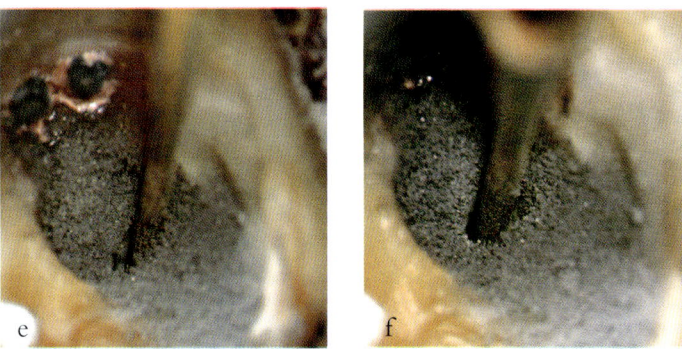

Fig 7-12 (e) Insertion of a diamond-coated tip to remove post material. (f) Ultrasonic vibration disrupts the post, producing a grey powder.

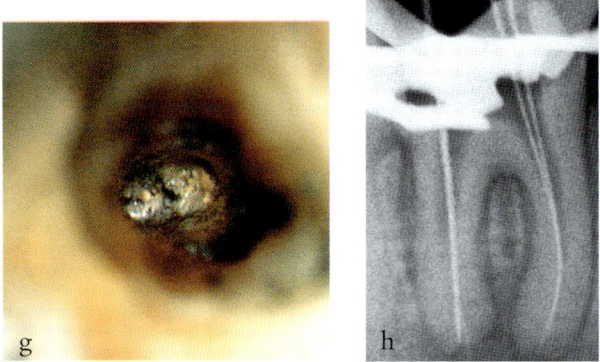

Fig 7-12 (g) Complete removal of the post. (h) The working length is reached after coronal and middle -third debridement.

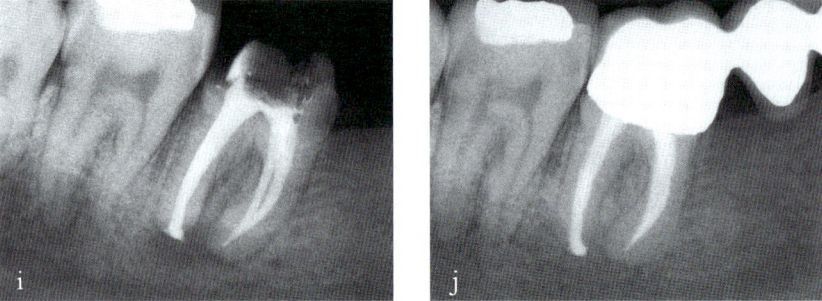

Fig 7-12 (i) Final obturation. (j) Three-year follow-up showing periapical healing.

Occasionally, it is apparent that the adhesive link between post and root canal wall is weak, and light vibrations may be all that is necessary to decement the post; a rare but pleasing situation (Fig 7-13a-h). The likely pool of hard cement at the base of the post-channel should, however, not be forgotten, and will need to be disrupted if entry to the apical part of the root is planned.

After the post has been removed, the walls of the post-channel should be carefully inspected, and ultrasonics used judiciously to remove remnants of composite cement. This is important not only to avoid inadvertent dislodgement and blocking of the canal during endodontic retreatment, but also to ensure a clean surface for subsequent rebonding after the completion of endodontic retreatment.

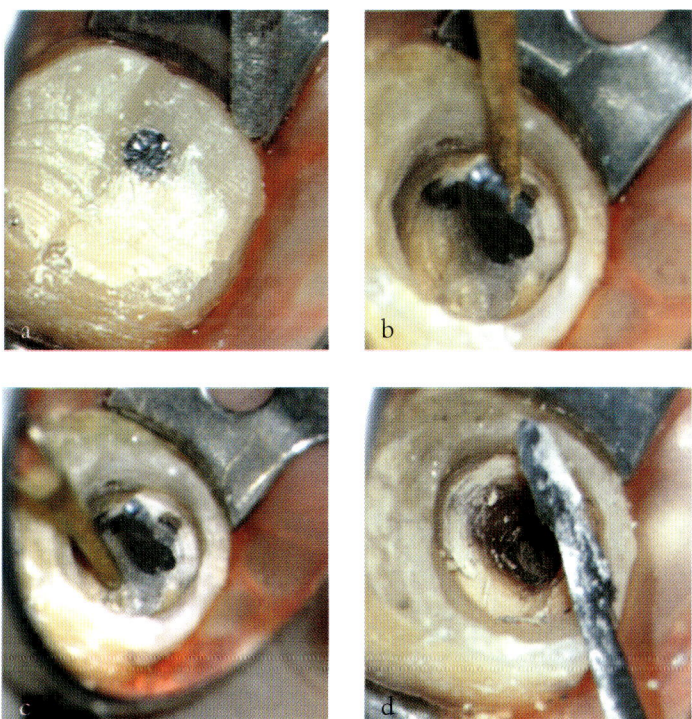

Fig 7-13 (a) A composite reconstruction to be removed with diamond-coated ultrasonic tips. (b) and (c) Working carefully around the post may helpfully weaken the bond with the dentinal substrate. (d) Judicious cutting might lead to complete removal of the intact post: note the luting agent around the post (continued over page).

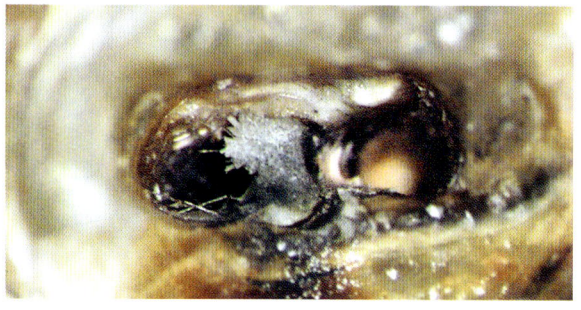

Fig 7-13 (e) A fibre post emerging from a premolar.

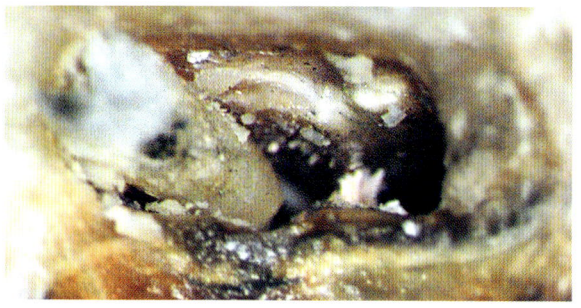

Fig 7-13 (f) Light, brief, intermittent touches with ultrasonic diamond-coated tips may remove the post intact.

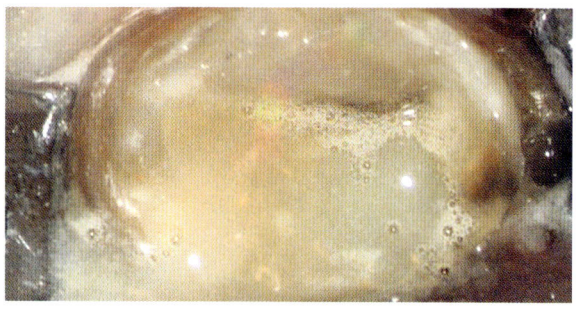

Fig 7-13 (g) Copious drainage from the canal following removal of the post.

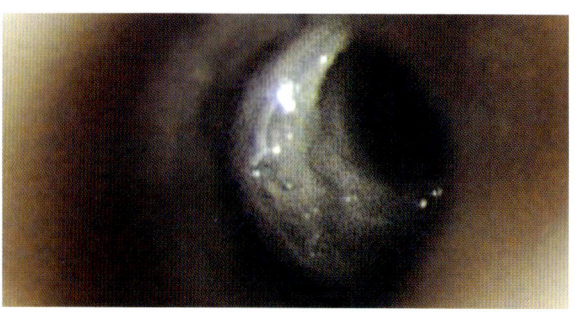

Fig 7-13 (h) All debris should be removed from canal walls with ultrasonics, using featherlight operating touches.

After the removal of the fibre post, the post's space will also be inspected to exclude the presence of root perforations. If a root perforation is present, the prognosis is less favourable and is dependent on the size and the time elapsed from the time of perforation. New materials such as mineral trioxide aggregate (MTA) have been employed to internally repair perforations and are widely trusted for effective repairs.

Endodontic retreatment may then follow in the usual way, with:
• further, light root canal preparation and irrigation to eliminate infection
• root canal filling and cut-back for optimal post-space.

The tooth may then receive a new bonded restoration.

Further Reading

Clark D. The operating microscope and ultrasonics; a perfect marriage. Dentistry Today 2004;23:78–81.

de Rijk WG. Removal of fibre posts from endodontically treated teeth. Am J D 2000;13:19B–21B.

Garcia A. Dental magnification: a clear view of the present and a close-up view of the future. Compendium of Continuing Education in Dentistry 2005;26:459–463.

Gesi A, Magnolfi S, Goracci C, Ferrari M. Comparison of two techniques for removing fibre posts. J Endod 2003;29:580–582.

Kim S. Principles of endodontic microsurgery. Dent Clin North Am 1997;41:481–497.

Kinomoto Y, Takeshige F, Hayashi M, Ebisu S. Optimal positioning for a dental operating microscope during nonsurgical endodontics. J Endod 2004;30:860–862.

Schwarze T, Baethge C, Stecher T, Geurtsen W. Identification of second canals in the mesiobuccal root of maxillary first and second molars using magnifying loupes or an operating microscope. Aust Endod J 2002;28:57–60.

Tsesis I, Rosen E, Schwartz-Arad D, Fuss Z. Retrospective evaluation of surgical endodontic treatment: traditional versus modern technique. J Endod 2006;32:412–416.

Chapter 8
The Restorability of Broken Down Teeth: the Decision-making Process

Aim

To discuss the factors which must be considered when assessing the restorability and managing the restoration of severely compromised teeth.

Outcome

At the end of this chapter, the reader should be able to make the decision when to restore the compromised tooth, and when to extract and consider options for replacement.

Objectives of Restoring a Severely Compromised Tooth
1. To promote tooth survival.
2. To restore pain-free function.
3. To protect the remaining tooth structure against further carious and non-carious tissue loss.
4. To provide occlusal stability and proximal contacts with adjacent teeth.
5. To provide optimal aesthetics.
6. To promote health in the marginal periodontal tissues.
7. To promote periapical health.

Following completion of the restorative treatment, the tooth should be able to withstand functional loads. The prognosis of the tooth is affected by a number of factors including the quality of the root canal treatment, the quality and quantity of the remaining coronal tooth structure, the avoidance of iatrogenic accidents such as perforation during post-space preparation, and the physical characteristics and fit of the core and the definitive restoration (Fig 8-1).

Restoration of Compromised Teeth

Optimal restorative management of the compromised tooth can only be achieved by making a systematic and thorough assessment of the tooth, within the context of the dentition, the supporting structures and the patient as a whole.

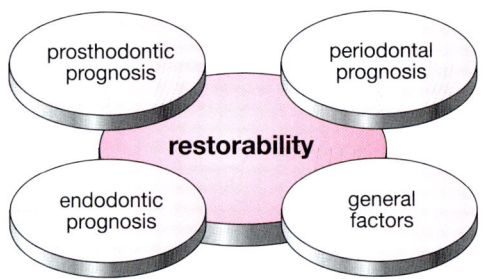

Fig 8-1 Factors affecting the restorability of a root canal treated tooth.

By completing a thorough clinical and radiographic examination, the restorability and overall prognosis of the tooth can be determined. These findings can then be presented to the patient, enabling an informed decision on the best way forward, based on the patient's expectations, motivation, time and financial constraints. The ultimate decision to restore or extract a severely compromised tooth must be dictated by informed patient choice. It is the responsibility of the dental professional to advise the patient of the treatment options, their relative prognosis and cost.

Many of the factors that are important in deciding whether or not to restore a tooth are also important when considering options for replacement if the tooth is lost. In addition, the status of the neighbouring teeth may be a very important consideration in deciding the best option for the patient.

Of course, every patient is different and this must be appreciated when treatment planning decisions are made. There are some patients who may be willing to go to almost any length in the hope of holding on to a tooth, even if the prognosis is acknowledged to be guarded. Alternatively, some patients may be reluctant to embark on any complex work, or wish only to invest in options which they consider to be predictable.

The discussions and the consent to proceed with a particular option should be recorded in the patient's notes. Written consent may be considered necessary in some instances.

Prognosis

Determining the prognosis of a tooth to be restored necessitates that a number of factors are considered, including the:

- **Prosthodontic prognosis**
- **Periodontal prognosis**
- **Endodontic prognosis**
- **Relevant general factors.**

Prosthodontic Prognosis

Key considerations include the:
- remaining sound coronal tooth structure
- presence or absence of fractures
- need to crown the tooth to protect against fracture
- ability to develop coronal seal
- ability to obtain ferrule protection
- occlusal factors
- ability to obtain satisfactory aesthetics.

Remaining Coronal Tooth Structure
The single most important factor influencing the prosthodontic prognosis is the amount of remaining sound coronal tooth structure. This tooth substance provides retention, resistance and a substrate for adhesion between the tooth and the restoration.

To assess the prognosis of a tooth, all restorations and any residual caries must be removed to allow inspection of the remaining tooth structure. A decision regarding the presence of adequate restorable coronal tooth structure can only be made once all the relevant information has been collected and carefully considered.

Presence of Fractures
The detection of any fractures in the remaining tooth structure is of paramount importance. A fracture may have a massive impact on the prognosis of the tooth. In addition to being a point of weakness in the tooth, fractures are a potential pathway for bacterial ingress into the root canal system and the marginal periodontium. Hence, a fracture can contribute to prosthodontic, periodontal and endodontic failure.

A fracture can be either complete or incomplete. Complete fractures are by definition obvious. Identifying incomplete fractures can be a diagnostic challenge. Fractures can be classified according to their location in the tooth:

- crown fracture – with or without pulpal involvement
- combined crown/root fracture
- isolated root fracture.

Crown Fracture

Crown fractures are seen fairly commonly, and may present in either restored or unrestored teeth. The clinical presentation may be as subtle as some crazing of the enamel, and as obvious as complete fracture and separation of a cusp or tooth wall. Teeth which have been heavily filled or root canal treated are more prone to developing fractures, but catastrophic fractures are occasionally seen in the sound, intact teeth of patients who parafunction. Some teeth may exhibit several fracture lines in different planes, in particular around a large restoration. Fractures can be considered as oblique or vertical in orientation. Vertical fractures usually present in a mesiodistal plane, running from one marginal ridge to another. Oblique fractures tend to occur at the fulcrum point adjacent to the base of a restoration. Vertical fractures may be more likely to result in an unrestorable outcome than other types of fracture.

There is an increased risk of developing tooth fractures with age. This may be related to the cumulative effects of caries, restorative intervention, and continued cyclical loading over years of function. A change in the composition and structure of dentine with age may also play some role in the development of fractures. Impact trauma may be an additional cause in a number of tooth fractures.

The diagnosis of a fractured tooth can, at times, be difficult, as the patient may complain of vague and poorly localised symptoms. The site, depth and completeness of a fracture is probably critical in dictating the type and level of pain. It is important to remember that the symptoms may be very different for fractures between vital and non-vital or root canal treated teeth. The symptoms experienced in fractured vital teeth are related to the effects of hydrodynamic fluid movement in the dentinal tubules and pulp. These pulpal symptoms will obviously not occur in teeth with non-vital pulps. Fractures in root canal treated teeth may only cause symptoms at a late stage, or if the fracture involves the root canal system or periodontal ligament.

Some of the key clinical features of fractured teeth are listed below, together with some clinical investigations which may be used to aid in the diagnosis of a root fracture (Fig 8-2).

Crown Fracture

Symptoms
- pain may be poorly localised or vague
- pain on biting, normally short-lived in duration
- sensitivity to thermal stimuli, usually cold
- symptoms of pulpitis may develop with time
- root canal treated teeth may have few or no symptoms.

Clinical features
- fracture may be oblique or vertical
- heavily restored teeth may be more susceptible
- fracture may be more evident in patients who parafunction
- fracture may not be visible on outer surface of tooth
- crazing of the enamel
- clearly demarcated and stained fracture lines
- tenderness to percussion of individual cusps
- pain on release after biting on cotton wool or Tooth Slooth/Frac Finder
- possible increased response to thermal pulp testing, usually cold.

Diagnosis

Clinical
- direct visualisation – may be aided with magnification
- removal of restoration to allow clear inspection of cavity
- transillumination – light will not cross an air-filled gap
- application of indicator dyes such as methylene blue
- individual percussion of cusps
- cotton wool roll, pain may be caused on release after biting
- symptom reproducers, e.g. Tooth Slooth
- thermal vitality testing, usually cold, e.g. Endofrost.

Radiographic
- unlikely to prove conclusive for coronal fractures alone
- extensive buccolingual fracture may be detected
- may be more important in excluding other causes of pain.

Management
Probably the two most important considerations when dealing with a fractured tooth are, to what extent the fracture will influence the restorability of the tooth, and whether the fracture extends to involve the pulp.

A supragingival fracture should not affect the prognosis significantly, unless there is a severe lack of coronal tooth structure. Restoration may be as simple as an adhesive cusp replacement restoration. Conversely, a subgingival fracture may render the tooth unrestorable, unless crown lengthening or rapid orthodontic extrusion are possible.

Pulpal involvement of the fracture will necessitate root canal treatment prior to definitive restoration. It is important, however, to establish that the fracture does not extend through the floor of the pulp chamber or into the root canals. Teeth which present with fractures which involve the floor of the pulp chamber or root canals have an uncertain prognosis. It may be impossible to tell whether the fracture is incomplete or complete and, hence, ensuring a bacterial seal with the root canal treatment cannot be achieved predictably. Even in those instances where the root fracture is incomplete on access, there is a very high possibility of propagating the fracture while carrying out the endodontic treatment. As a result, patients should be advised that teeth demonstrating fractures involving the pulp carry a poor or hopeless prognosis.

Root Fracture

Root fracture can occur as a continuation of a coronal fracture or in isolation. Once a fracture involves the periodontal ligament, the nature and severity of the patient's symptoms may change significantly (see below). The patient is more likely to complain of increased pain on biting, and this will generally be more easily localised and diagnosed. Unfortunately, periodontal ligament involvement of a fracture is an indicator of poor prognosis.

The causes of root fracture are the same as those that cause coronal fracture (i.e. physiological and pathological stresses), and teeth that have been root canal treated and restored with a post are most susceptible to root fracture. Post-restored teeth that are involved in excursive movements are especially at risk of fracture as a result of laterally applied loads. The iatrogenic causes of root fracture include root canal preparation and obturation, post cementation and post removal.

Root Fracture

Symptoms
- mild to moderate pain
- pain on mastication
- increased mobility
- sinus tract or swelling.

Clinical features
- typically seen in susceptible teeth, e.g. post-crowned teeth
- osseous defect adjacent to the fracture
- periodontal pocketing, classically a localised deep periodontal pocket not consistent with the general periodontal condition. Typically located bucally
- possible tenderness to percussion. More prolonged than that seen in crown fracture
- buccal or lingual tenderness to palpation
- sinus tract formation, soft-tissue swelling or erythema
- if present, a sinus tract is usually more coronal than typically seen with periapical disease; often coronal to the mucogingival junction
- increased mobility may be observed.

Clinical diagnosis
- direct visualisation, may be aided by gently probing and pulling back the gingivae adjacent to the fracture
- surgical visualisation
- identification of localised osseous defect
- direct visualisation of fracture line.

Radiographic diagnosis
- about 30% of root fractures can be diagnosed radiographically
- at least two different horizontally angled radiographs should be taken to aid diagnosis.

Key radiographic features include:
- hair-like fracture lines which may be detected in the dentine body
- separation of tooth fragments
- classical "halo" or J-shaped radiolucency, with bone loss around the peri-apex and continuous with the lateral root surface (Fig 8-2)
- bone loss on the lateral root surface similar to that of a periodontal defect.

Management
- fractured roots usually require extraction
- root resection may be possible in certain multi-rooted teeth.

Protection against Fracture
Clinical studies on the restoration of root canal treated teeth have shown that anterior teeth do not necessarily need to be restored with a crown. Even

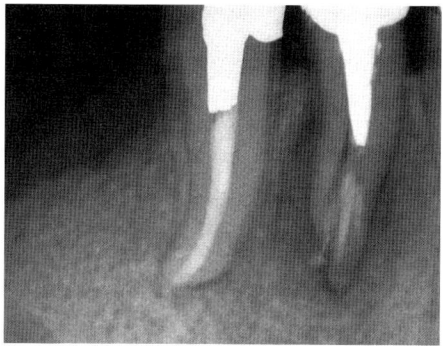

Fig 8-2 A root fracture in a mandibular first premolar restored using a cast post and crown.

quite extensive loss of proximal tissue in addition to the endodontic access does not necessarily weaken the tooth to the extent to warrant a crown. In fact, there is evidence to suggest that the tissue loss associated with crown preparation in such circumstances may irreversibly weaken the residual tooth substance to a damaging extent, predisposing to failure.

In the case of endodontically treated posterior teeth, the current best evidence indicates significantly longer tooth survival subsequent to the provision of a partial or full coverage cast restoration (Fig 8-3).

Premolars require careful assessment as the benefits of a full cuspal coverage restoration must be carefully balanced against the potentially destructive preparation of the tooth for a cast restoration.

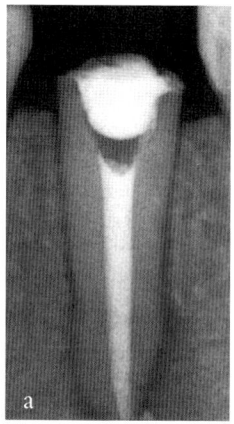
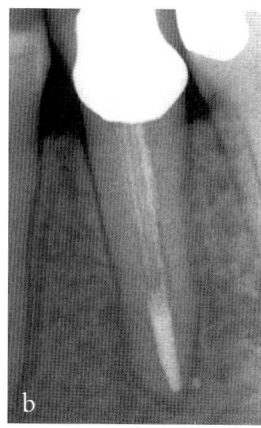

Fig 8-3 (a) A severely damaged mandibular premolar restored with a fibre post and a metal-ceramic crown. (b) A five-year recall radiograph.

Coronal Seal

Coronal restorations of poor quality have been regarded by some researchers as important pathways for the entry of micro-organisms and nutrient fluids into teeth, with compromising effects on even well-conducted root canal treatments.

The evidence is far from clear, with some reports claiming that the quality of the coronal restoration may be just as important to periapical health as the quality of the root canal treatment. Conversely, other reports suggest that teeth which have been root canal treated to a high standard are unlikely to develop apical periodontitis even when the coronal restoration has suffered gross leakage or been missing for a prolonged period of time. The conclusion to be drawn from the current best evidence is that the coronal seal protects against secondary caries, and plays some role in endodontic outcome and tooth survival. It is recommended, therefore, that strenuous efforts be made to provide sealing of provisional and permanent restorations with a good marginal seal to guard the root canal system from microbial and fluid entry.

Ferrule Effect

The ability to obtain a ferrule effect is pivotal to the success of any extracoronal restoration, irrelevant of the core that has been placed (see Chapter 3). Core fracture, post decementation or root fracture are the usual adverse consequences of inadequate or absent ferrule preparation. The precise extent of an adequate ferrule remains contentious, with the complete envelopment of at least 2 mm of coronal tooth tissue regarded as optimal. In many circumstances, this may not be possible, but at least 1 mm may be the lower limit, beyond which serious questions must be asked about the prognosis of the tooth. In addition to the ferrule being of adequate height, the ring of tissue which is enveloped by the extracoronal restoration must be of sufficient thickness for structural durability.

Current research data are not very helpful in this respect, but a minimum of 1 mm thickness is widely regarded as necessary to resist the lateral forces placed on the restored tooth. Ideally, the ferrule should be continuous around the entire circumference of the tooth.

Any ferrule should be considered in the context of the individual case, with regard to the occlusion and the quality and nature of the post and core in that case. Contemporary adhesive techniques may allow thinner sections of coronal tissue to be preserved in a way that is not possible with traditional methods.

Suitability for a post

If the decision has been made that a post is necessary to restore the tooth to function, then certain considerations must be made. These include:

- *Crown/post ratio*

Various researchers have demonstrated higher success rates for posts that are equal to or greater in length than the clinical crown.

- *Diameter of the root*

A post which is a third or less of the diameter of the root has been shown to be associated with a lower probability of root fracture.

- *Curvature of root canals*

The curvature of the chosen root canals must be considered and it follows that straighter canals carry a lower risk of iatrogenic perforation during post-space preparation. Equally, care should be exercised in the post-space preparation of roots with marked concavities.

Occlusal Factors

Occlusal factors may be of paramount importance in assessing the prosthodontic prognosis of a compromised tooth. Tooth location, the number of teeth present, heavy guidance, the presence of deflective contacts or interferences, and evidence of wear, mobility or repeated fracture of the restored and adjacent or opposing teeth may alert the dentist that long-term survival of the restoration may be compromised.

There is no doubt that the presence of a guiding contact in excursive movements is unfavourable to the prosthodontic prognosis of a tooth. Conversely, a patient who has a compromised tooth which is clear of any excursive contacts may have a better chance of tooth survival subsequent to complex restorative treatment.

There is also no doubt that parafunctional activity affects the predictability of all aspects of restorative dentistry, and nowhere is this more important than with the restoration of the broken down tooth. Broken down teeth cannot be successfully restored in patients who parafunction unless they are kept free from occlusal contact or if there is enough coronal tooth structure to withstand the atypical forces which may come to bear. Restorations in such patients must be as retentive as possible, and at the same time reinforce the teeth rather than weaken them. Patients who parafunction may also benefit from some form of protective occlusal appliance.

Aesthetic Factors

In addition to restoring function, the final restoration should meet the realistic aesthetic expectations of the patient. When considering the final aesthetic outcome of the restoration, the clinician must consider the effect that the treatment may have on the appearance of the tooth. For example, if crown lengthening is required to expose adequate coronal tooth tissue to provide a ferrule, the final aesthetic result may be unacceptable to the patient. However, the same patient may also find the aesthetics of a conventional bridge to replace the tooth unsatisfactory.

Periodontal Prognosis

Key considerations include:
- oral hygiene and patient motivation
- gingival health and pocketing
- bony support
- root length and anatomy.

Once the prosthodontic assessment has been completed, and the clinician is satisfied that the coronal tooth structure can be restored predictably, the periodontal prognosis of the tooth must be ascertained (Fig 8-4).

Loss of attachment and bone loss must be considered when assessing the periodontal prognosis and overall restorability of a tooth. Increased mobility, advanced recession or furcation involvement may preclude predictable restoration. An isolated area of deep pocketing in an otherwise periodontally sound dentition may raise the question of a longitudinal root fracture, which usually carries a hopeless prognosis.

If, despite advanced periodontal disease, a patient is still keen to retain a compromised tooth, periodontal treatment must be carried out and the healing response assessed prior to the construction of any definitive restoration. Of course, successful periodontal therapy is dependent on the patient being highly motivated to secure and maintain an optimal level of oral hygiene, and with the understanding that the introduction of complex restorations may increase the demands for stringent maintenance.

Occasionally, due to extensive caries, subgingival restorative margins, or an attempt to maximise retention, crown margins encroach on the biological width. Such margins are associated with gingival inflammation, loss of attachment and localised periodontal destruction (Fig 8-5). To avoid these

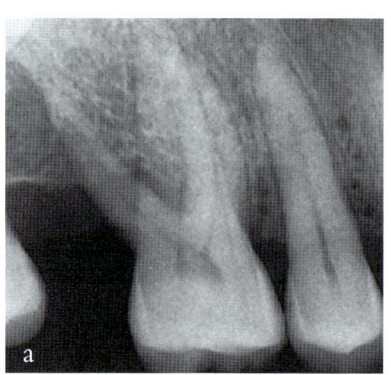

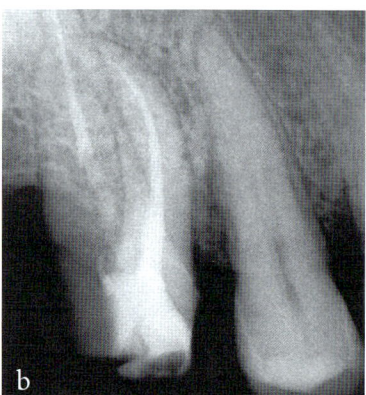

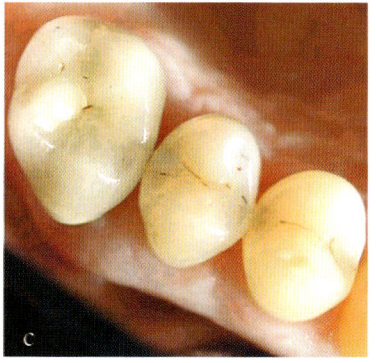

Fig 8-4 The maxillary first molar shows furcation involvement between the distal and palatal root (a). After the resection of the distal root and the restoration using a fibre post and composite (b). The tooth was restored with a metal-ceramic crown (c).

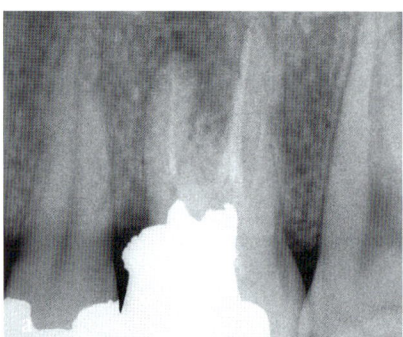

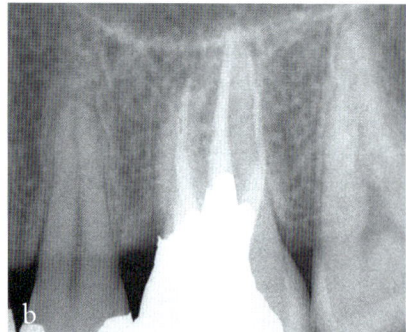

Fig 8-5 The amalgam restoration of the maxillary first molar is impinging on the biological width (a). The tooth shows a periapical radiolucency and needs retreatment. At the five-year recall, the radiolucency has healed but the new amalgam restoration is still impinging on the biological width.

undesirable consequences, crown margins should wherever possible be placed supragingivally. As well as avoiding disruption to the biological width, keeping the restorative margins supragingivally allows optimal maintenance and plaque control.

However, aesthetic demands may rule out supragingival margin placement, and an agreed compromise may be needed to place the margins at or near the level of the gingival sulcus. If this is not possible, then crown lengthening or rapid orthodontic extrusion may be considered (see Chapter 3). If neither of these treatment options is feasible, and the patient's aesthetic expectations cannot be met without significant periodontal compromise, the restorative prognosis should be considered as poor.

Crown Lengthening

Crown lengthening should not be considered in patients who have active periodontal disease or poor oral hygiene/motivation and those who have caries or restorative margins which extend into the furcation area of the tooth. When considering crown lengthening procedures, it is imperative to remember that bone removal is necessary in order to achieve the desired lengthening and at the same time maintain the biological width. Procedures which involve soft tissue manipulation alone are not considered proper crown lengthening. The effect of bone removal on the overall prognosis of the tooth should be considered prior to embarking on treatment. If crown lengthening is required, its impact on the final aesthetic result must also be evaluated fully.

Perio–endo Lesions

The possibility of a combined perio-endo lesion should not be overlooked when assessing the compromised tooth. It occurs in teeth which exhibit both marginal attachment loss and apical periodontitis. Marginal periodontitis may advance apically to devitalise a pulp, in which case the prognosis is usually hopeless. Alternatively, a periapical lesion of endodontic origin may extend coronally along the root surface to communicate with the periodontal pocket. In this situation, the endodontic component of the lesion should fully heal after successful root canal treatment. What initially presented as a very deep probing defect should rapidly become less severe. Further periodontal care is then required to manage the residual periodontal lesion. Periodontal-endodontic lesions may be classified in many ways, but the important message is that the endodontic care should preceed any deep periodontal instrumentation. The overall prognosis for the tooth does rely, however, on successful endodontic and periodontal care.

Endodontic Prognosis

Key considerations include:
• access to treat the tooth
• ability to isolate the tooth
• ability to identify all root canals
• ability to negotiate, shape, clean and fill all canals to length (curvature, calcification).

The prognosis of root canal treatment in relation to preoperative pulpal and periradicular status and technical outcome is summarised in Fig 8-6.

Determinants of Endodontic Success

Endodontic success is dependent on the ability to eliminate microbial infection from the root canal system and prevent recolonisation or reactivation by leakage of nutrients through apical, lateral and coronal pathways. The technical factors which are most likely to compromise treatment are limited access, inability to isolate the tooth, and inability to identify and negotiate all canals to length (e.g. as a result of internal calcification or root curvature).

Endodontic success can be defined in a variety of ways, from painless function to complete resolution of periapical inflammation. Established guidelines recommend that root canal treated teeth are monitored for up to four years

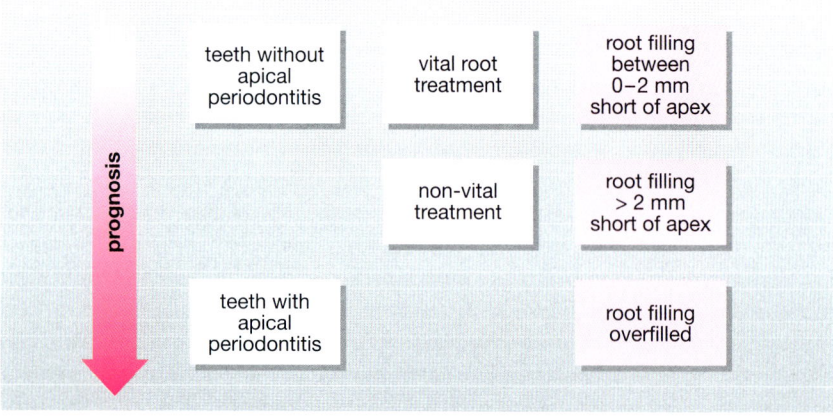

Fig 8-6 The prognosis of root canal treatment in relation to preoperative pulpal and periradicular status and technical outcome.

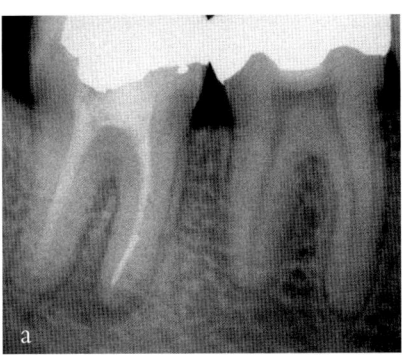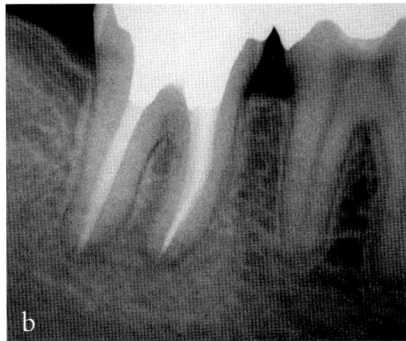

Fig 8-7 Tooth 47 shows a periapical radiolucency associated with both roots. A fractured instrument is evident in the apical region of the mesial root (a). The six-month recall shows initial healing.

before "success" or "failure" can be established, and emphasise the clinical and radiographic resolution of endodontic disease. Although radiographic lesions may take significantly longer than this to fully heal, a healing response can often be inferred sooner (Fig 8-7). The minimum period recommended to assess clinical and radiographic healing is one year post-treatment.

Where a sealing and protective coronal restoration is to be provided at the same visit, or shortly after the root canal treatment, a decision must be made on prognosis without the benefit of observing healing. There is strong evidence that root canal treatment is most successful in teeth which are root canal treated before apical periodontitis is evident. Success rates in such circumstances can be as high as 95%. In cases in which apical periodontitis is established, successful treatment may be anticipated in a smaller percentage, perhaps 80–90% of cases.

In technical terms, successful root canal treatment appears to be strongly associated with homogeneous root fillings which extend to within 0–2 mm of the root-end and with no significant extrusion of material into the periapical tissues. The slowest healing responses are seen in teeth with over-extended root fillings (Fig 8-8).

When the restoration of a root treated tooth requires post placement, a minimum of 4–5 mm of well-condensed root filling should be present below the post to provide an apical seal. In addition, efforts should be made to ensure that the post is well fitting, and so does not act as a pathway for microleakage.

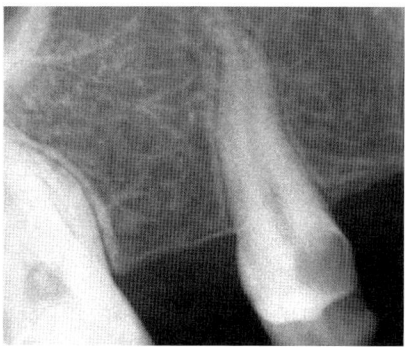 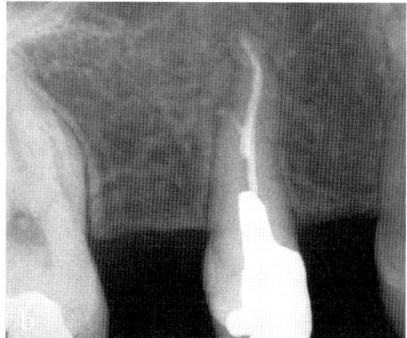

Fig 8-8 The second maxillary premolar shows caries communicating with the pulp chamber and a periapical radiolucency (a). The one-year recall shows an initial healing of the periapical radiolucency, but a new radiolucency is now associated with an extrusion of root filling material into the periodontal space via a lateral canal.

Therefore, when considering the potential length of a post, allowance must be made to conserve enough root filling to allow an adequate apical seal.

The post should be as well adapted as possible with the coronal extent of the root filling to preclude an undesirable void in the canal. In addition, careful assessment of the canal's suitability for post placement should be made to reduce the risk of iatrogenic errors during post-space preparation.

Iatrogenic Factors
The influence of iatrogenic factors on endodontic prognosis cannot be excluded when considering endodontic prognosis. Technical difficulties and operational mishaps can reduce the likelihood of success in endodontic treatment. Reminding ourselves that root canal treatment is about eliminating micro-organisms and preventing their recurrence, any procedural difficulties which compromise disinfection and final seal may significantly compromise the healing outcome.

Iatrogenic factors preventing optimal disinfection of the root canal system include:
- missed canal(s)
- poor asepsis and lack of use of appropriate irrigants
- inadequate apical preparation/taper preventing optimal irrigant delivery
- inability to instrument and clean the full length of the root canal due to ledging, obstructions of other causes (e.g. dental debris, fractured instruments).

The impact of these factors may be greater in teeth with established intracanal infection and apical periodontitis than in those without heavy microbial contamination.

Iatrogenic factors contributing to potential reinfection of the root canal system include:
- absent or under-extended root fillings
- poorly condensed root fillings
- root perforations and fractures
- suboptimal coronal seal following endodontic treatment.

If any of the above situations are present in a tooth, there is a potential pathway for microbial or nutrient fluid penetration of the root canal system following treatment. Unfilled spaces within this system may provide a favourable environment for endodontic pathogens to colonise. Iatrogenic perforations are an unfortunate complication of root canal treatment. These can include perforations of the pulp chamber floor, strip perforations of the root canal or even perforations which are caused during post-space preparation. A perforation provides a clear and often large route for reinfection of the root canal system. Technically, the management of a perforation may be demanding, and the site, size and nature of the communication may complicate the ability to obtain a fluid- and microbe-tight seal. As a result, usually the prognosis of teeth with perforations must be regarded as unpredictable.

General Factors

Key considerations include:
- access to dental care
- motivation to preserve teeth
- financial and time consequences of complex treatment
- the need for, and compliance with, stringent maintenance.

Difficulties with mobility and access to the dental surgery, the impracticality of domiciliary care, or barriers created by multiple, long journeys for complex care may modulate treatment-planning decisions in some circumstances. Equally, long treatment sessions may be intolerable for some patients, regardless of their motivation to save their teeth, and treatment plans may need to be modified accordingly.

Patient motivation is imperative, not just at the point of treatment delivery, but also in long-term maintenance. For example, stringent daily plaque control and regular visits to the dental hygienist may be essential following complex tooth restoration and related treatment.

There may be instances where an unmotivated patient demands extensive restorative care. Patients who are unable to demonstrate an adequate level of oral hygiene or alter lifestyle factors such as their dietary or smoking habits, despite being given appropriate advice or instruction, may not be good candidates for complex restorative treatment. It is very important not to be coerced into providing treatment which is doomed to failure. In such circumstances, it is important to discuss the aetiology of treatment failure in plain terms, often with clear illustrations, so that the concerns of the dentist are known and an agreed plan can be reached.

The relative costs of all the treatment options must be conveyed to the patient. These should include not only the immediate, direct costs, but also the future costs of maintenance or managing failure. A clear understanding of prognosis is essential if patients are to understand the risk of treatment failure, and the costs of remedial treatment. This is important especially in cases in which the patient is inclined to opt for a treatment option which has a lesser prognosis.

A detailed consideration of all relevant issues is important in decision-making for the compromised tooth, ensuring awareness of risks and benefits, and encouraging rational decision-making. The stepwise assessment process is summarised in Fig 8-9.

Alternative Options

The alternative to restoring the compromised tooth is to extract the tooth and then restore the gap with an implant, bridge or denture as follows:
- extraction with no prosthetic replacement
- implant placement
- bridge placement – conventional and minimal preparation, resin-bonded
- removable partial denture.

Extraction
This may be of special concern if the tooth is in an aesthetic region. The isolated loss of a single posterior tooth is unlikely to compromise masticatory function in most patients. The possible undesirable consequences of unrestored tooth loss, including tipping and over-eruption of adjacent teeth, should be discussed, as such consequences may complicate prosthodontic efforts at a later date.

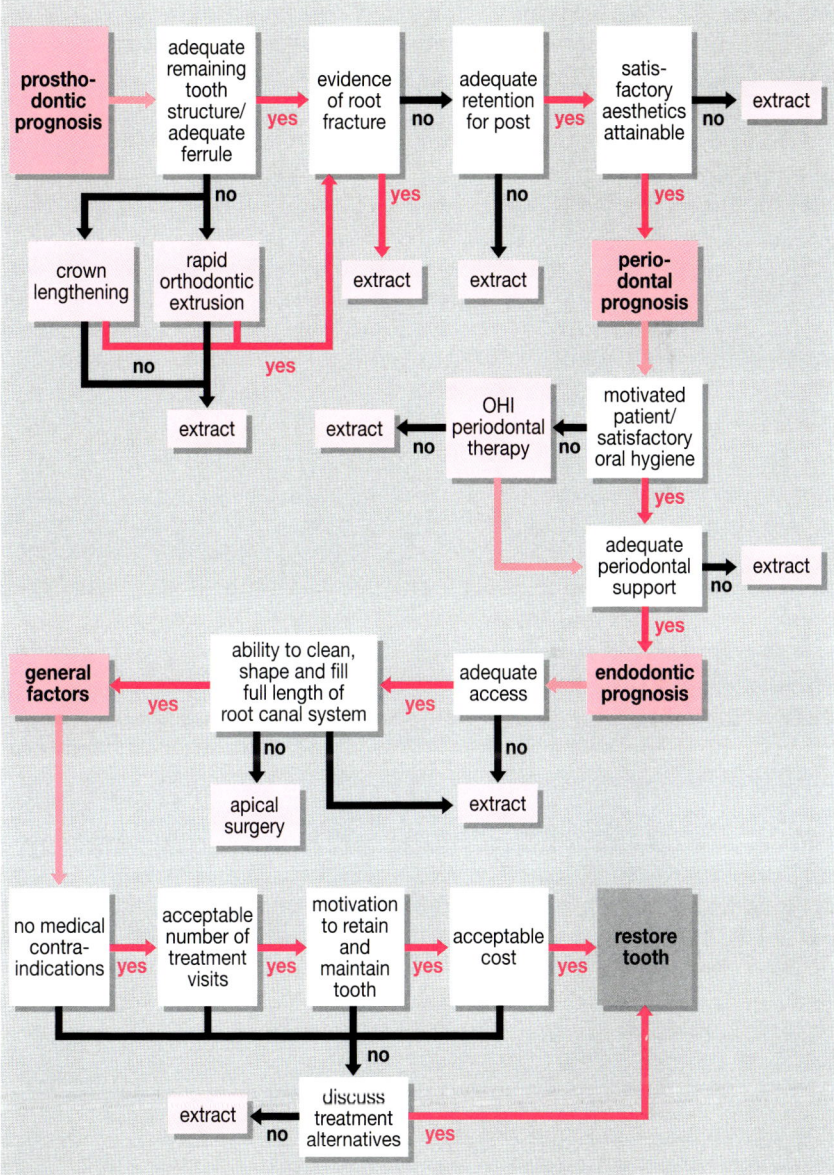

Fig 8-9 Factors involved in the assessment and treatment planning of the compromised tooth.

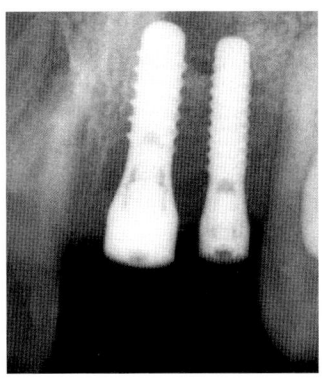

Fig 8-10 Implants placed for the replacement of a maxillary central and lateral incisor.

Implant Placement

The increasing use of osseo-integrated implants has probably been one of the most exciting developments in dentistry in recent times. The survival of implants is documented to be greater than 90% over 15 years. With few exceptions, dental implants are the ideal means of restoring single-unit spaces. They offer a highly predictable, fully integrated and fixed restoration without involvement of the adjacent teeth (Fig 8-10).

Unfortunately, there are some practitioners who, when discussing treatment outcomes with patients, quote low success rates for endodontic treatment and subsequent restoration compared with implant placement. These statements are made without appreciating that outcome data for endodontic and implant treatments are based generally on different definitions of "success".

Therefore, direct comparison of headline figures can be misleading. The predictability and role of implants as a restorative option is beyond question, but root canal treatment and subsequent restoration can also lead to a favourable clinical outcome.

Traditionally, the criteria for defining endodontic success were set at a high level, based on histological and radiographic parameters. By contrast, the success of an implant treatment is usually defined as functional survival of the implant fixture. Evaluation criteria for implants usually allow bone loss of up to 0.2 mm per annum around fixtures without questioning success (Fig 8-11), whereas bone loss in relation to a root-filled tooth would be an indication of failure.

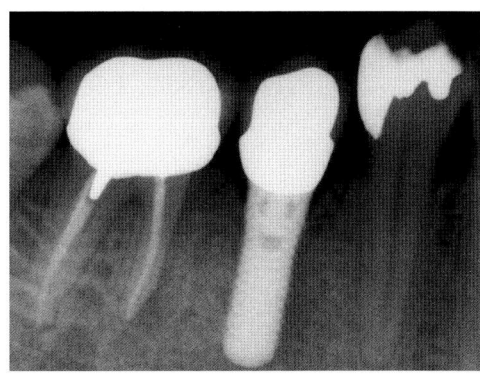

Fig 8-11 Normally, a moderate bone loss around an implant fixture is not regarded as failure.

Recent studies focusing on functional survival of root canal treated teeth have shown outcomes comparable to those of implant treatment.

In addition to the stringent success criteria used in endodontic outcome studies, it is also important to consider the definition of failure. In most endodontic studies, if the initial root canal treatment does not fully heal the periapical lesion, the case is considered a failure. This does not mean, however, that the tooth is no longer surviving in function or that there are no options for further non-surgical or surgical treatment for its preservation, should they be necessary (Fig 8-10).

A key point of differentiation; root treatment acts to retain what is there while implantology aims to restore what is missing. Therefore, endodontic treatment with a lesser prognosis may be accepted in an attempt to preserve what is already there.

Limitations of implants
Implant surgery is able to overcome most clinical problems, but there are still situations where involved preparatory surgery may be necessary prior to implant placement. Sinus lifts, nerve repositioning procedures and bone grafts may be carried out of course, but these additional procedures should not be forgotten about when discussing treatment options with patients.

Despite the rapid advances in implant dentistry, there is still a relatively high morbidity of these restorations in patients who parafunction. As this group of patients is becoming more prevalent, it is important to remember that it may not always be possible to consider implant-retained prostheses as a treatment option. Furthermore, the emotional consideration of implant surgery is significant, and this is not acknowledged in any outcome studies. The retention of the natural dentition is important to most patients, and the effects of tooth loss, implant surgery and often a period of time without a fixed prosthesis must be considered when evaluating treatment modalities.

Bridges

If it is not possible to replace a missing tooth with an implant, a fixed-bridge alternative may be considered. There are two main approaches:

- conventional fixed bridgework
- minimal preparation, resin-bonded bridgework.

Conventional fixed bridge

The survival rate of well-maintained conventional bridgework may be as high as 74% after 15 years. Of course, variations in design, quality and quantity of abutment teeth and pontics, arch position and occlusion may significantly influence the prognosis of each individual case.

The conventional fixed bridge is a complex restoration, requiring a high standard of diagnosis, treatment planning and clinical execution in order to obtain success. Construction of a conventional fixed bridge involves preparing adjacent teeth to receive full or partial coverage extracoronal restorations. As a consequence, bridge preparation requires significant coronal dentine removal, which will weaken abutment teeth significantly, in particular, when internal losses have already occurred in previous operative dentistry and root canal treatment.

In addition, it must be borne in mind that the preparation of teeth with vital pulps may result in short- or long-term pulp necrosis. It is imperative that the pulpal and periapical health of the abutment teeth is established prior to conventional bridge preparation. If complex fixed bridgework is to be carried out on teeth where pulpal and periapical health cannot be confidently determined as healthy, then these teeth should be root canal treated prior to bridgework.

Bridge preparation in itself may lead to a tooth which has an uncertain pulpal status to flare-up. It may also be necessary to electively root canal treat teeth where significant removal of coronal tooth structure is necessary, for example where a tilted molar requires "uprighting" to act as a bridge abutment.

Sometimes, it may be wrongly assumed that because a tooth is root canal treated, heavily restored and in need of a crown, it is a good candidate as a bridge abutment. It may be felt that there is good justification in taking a bur to heavily filled teeth but, in reality, they are often unreliable bridge abutments, given the weakening caused by tooth tissue loss and the risks of cyclical loading with functional forces in excess of those placed on a single-unit restoration. In particular, there is evidence to suggest that teeth restored with post-retained cores are the least favourable teeth to act as bridge abutments.

In addition to the direct consequences of tooth preparation, the following factors should be considered:
- *Functional loading* – By placing a conventional bridge, functional loads on the abutment teeth are increased. This effect may accelerate crack propagation and cyclical fatigue of abutment teeth.
- *Caries and periodontal disease* – Following placement of a conventional bridge, there is an increased risk of localised periodontal disease and secondary caries. Even the best restoration margin may present opportunities for plaque accumulation, and all patients receiving fixed bridgework should enter a planned maintenance regime.
- *Lack of retrievability* – This is probably the biggest problem with conventional bridges. If an abutment develops a problem such as caries, periodontal disease, core decementation or fracture, then the entire bridge usually needs to be removed. The bridge may also require removal if one of the abutment teeth becomes non-vital, or if apical periodontitis develops on a root canal treated abutment tooth. Therefore, the management of complications with abutment teeth is invariably complicated.

Minimal preparation resin-bonded bridgework
Research suggests that the survival rate of resin-retained bridges approaches 80% over four years. The most common modality of failure is debonding from abutments.

Resin-bonded bridgework has significant advantages over conventional bridgework as it requires minimal tooth preparation and is usually of cantilever design, involving only one abutment. Therefore, the undesirable consequences of tooth preparation are minimised.

Although there is significantly less tooth tissue destruction than with a conventional bridge, there is still an increased risk of periodontal disease and recurrent caries. In addition, if two abutment teeth are used for a resin-retained bridge, there is a risk of one wing debonding with the development of caries beneath the debonded wing. As the bridge is still retained by the other wing, caries may progress rapidly and to a significant degree before the patient becomes aware of the problem.

Debond – the most common mode of failure, is caused generally by poor case selection, absence of tooth preparation or poor bridge design. The occlusion may also play a decisive role; for example, debonding is a frequent complication when a resin-retained bridge is used to restore an anterior tooth, where there is a deep overbite. When replacing premolar and molar teeth, it is important that the retainer wings are designed to incorporate maximal wrap-around and cuspal coverage.

Removable Partial Denture

The advantages of a removable partial denture are its relative simplicity and that little, if any, tooth preparation is required.

However, patient acceptance of a removable partial denture may be poor. The removable prosthesis may be uncomfortable, encourage increased plaque levels, and food packing, and compromise mastication and speech. In addition, the patient may find the removable nature of the prosthesis functionally or socially unacceptable. It can, in certain cases, be difficult to obtain acceptable aesthetics with a partial denture.

Of course, there are instances where the removable partial denture is the most appropriate treatment option. Periodontally compromised abutment teeth can be retained with a well-designed removable prosthesis, while facilitating easy addition in the event of their loss. Teeth that have short clinical crowns or short root length may serve better as removable partial denture abutments than fixed bridge abutments. Removable partial dentures may also be useful in cases where there has been extensive tissue loss in an edentulous area.

When considering a partial denture as a treatment option, it is imperative that the patient is able to maintain a high standard of oral hygiene.

Conclusion

The decision to restore or extract a compromised tooth can only be determined after a thorough clinical and radiographic examination. This information may then be used to determine restorability in prosthodontic, periodontal, endodontic and aesthetic terms. Each element of the examination informs a view on the likely success of complex restorative treatment, which combined with information on other treatment options, helps the patient and dentist to reach a realistic treatment plan. A logical and structured assessment protocol, combined with an evaluation of patient motivation and aspirations, will ensure that the best treatment options are offered to each individual patient.

Further Reading

Ahlberg KF, Rowe AHR, Pitt Ford TR, Stock CJR, Leigh B. Consensus report of the European Society of Endodontology on quality guidelines for endodontic treatment. Int Endod J 1994;27:115–124.

Creugers NH, Kayser AF, van't Hof MA. A meta-analysis of durability data on conventional fixed bridges. Community Dent Oral Epidemiol 1994;: 448–452.

Djemal S, Setchell D, King P, Wickens J. Long-term survival characteristics of 832 resin-retained bridges and splints provided in a post-graduate teaching hospital between 1978 and 1993. J Oral Rehabil 1999;26:302–320.

Kojima K, Inamoto K, Nagamatsu K, Hara A, Nakata K, Morita I. Success rate of endodontic treatment of teeth with vital and non-vital pulps. A meta-analysis. Oral Surg Oral Med Oral Pathol 2004;97:95–99.

Sjögren U, Hägglund B, Sundqvist G, Wing K. Factors affecting the long-term results of endodontic treatment. J Endod 1990;16:498–504.

Tait CME, Ricketts DNJ, Higgins AJ. Restoration of the root-filled tooth: pre-operative assessment. Br Dent J 2005;:395–404.

Index

Quintessentials for General Dental Practitioners Series

in 50 volumes

Editor-in-Chief: Professor Nairn H F Wilson

The Quintessentials for General Dental Practitioners Series covers basic principles and key issues in all aspects of modern dental medicine. Each book can be read as a stand-alone volume or in conjunction with other books in the series.

Publication date, approximately

Clinical Practice, Editor: Nairn Wilson

Culturally Sensitive Oral Healthcare	available
Dental Erosion	available
Special Care Dentistry	available
Evidence Based Dentistry	Autumn 2007
Infection Control for the Dental Team	Winter 2007
Therapeutics and Medical Emergencies in the Everyday Clinical Practice of Dentistry	Winter 2007

Oral Surgery and Oral Medicine, Editor: John G Meechan

Practical Dental Local Anaesthesia	available
Practical Oral Medicine	available
Practical Conscious Sedation	available
Minor Oral Surgery in Dental Practice	available

Imaging, Editor: Keith Horner

Interpreting Dental Radiographs	available
Panoramic Radiology	available
21st Century Dental Imaging	available

Periodontology, Editor: Iain L C Chapple

Understanding Periodontal Diseases: Assessment and Diagnostic Procedures in Practice	available
Decision-Making for the Periodontal Team	available
Successful Periodontal Therapy – A Non-Surgical Approach	available
Periodontal Management of Children, Adolescents and Young Adults	available
Periodontal Medicine: A Window on the Body	available
Contemporary Periodontal Surgery – An Illustrated Guide to the Art Behind the Science	Autumn 2007

Endodontics, Editor: John M Whitworth

Rational Root Canal Treatment in Practice	available
Managing Endodontic Failure in Practice	available
Adhesive Restoration of Endodontically Treated Teeth	available

Prosthodontics, Editor: P Finbarr Allen

Teeth for Life for Older Adults	available
Complete Dentures – from Planning to Problem Solving	available
Removable Partial Dentures	available
Fixed Prosthodontics in Dental Practice	available
Occlusion: A Theoretical and Team Approach	Autumn 2007
Managing Orofacial Pain in Practice	Winter 2007

Operative Dentistry, Editor: Paul A Brunton

Decision-Making in Operative Dentistry	available
Aesthetic Dentistry	available
Communicating in Dental Practice	available
Indirect Restorations	available
Dental Bleaching	available
Choosing and Using Dental Materials	Autumn 2007
Composite Restorations in Posterior Teeth	Winter 2007

Paediatric Dentistry/Orthodontics, Editor: Marie Therese Hosey

Child Taming: How to Manage Children in Dental Practice	available
Paediatric Cariology	available
Treatment Planning for the Developing Dentition	available
Managing Dental Trauma in Practice	available

General Dentistry and Practice Management, Editor: Raj Rattan

The Business of Dentistry	available
Risk Management in General Dental Practice	available
Quality Matters: From Clinical Care to Customer Service	available
Practice Management for the Dental Team	Winter 2007

Dental Team, Editor: Mabel Slater

Team Players in Dentistry	Winter 2007

Implantology, Editor: Lloyd J Searson

Implantology in General Dental Practice	available

Quintessence Publishing Co. Ltd., London